Healthcare Changes and the Affordable Care Act

James S. Powers
Editor

Healthcare Changes and the Affordable Care Act

A Physician Call to Action

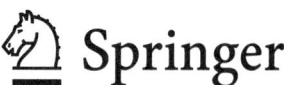

Editor
James S. Powers
Vanderbilt University School of Medicine
Nashville, TN, USA

ISBN 978-3-319-09509-7 ISBN 978-3-319-09510-3 (eBook)
DOI 10.1007/978-3-319-09510-3
Springer Cham Heidelberg New York Dordrecht London

Library of Congress Control Number: 2014951197

© Springer International Publishing Switzerland 2015
This work is subject to copyright. All rights are reserved by the Publisher, whether the whole or part of the material is concerned, specifically the rights of translation, reprinting, reuse of illustrations, recitation, broadcasting, reproduction on microfilms or in any other physical way, and transmission or information storage and retrieval, electronic adaptation, computer software, or by similar or dissimilar methodology now known or hereafter developed. Exempted from this legal reservation are brief excerpts in connection with reviews or scholarly analysis or material supplied specifically for the purpose of being entered and executed on a computer system, for exclusive use by the purchaser of the work. Duplication of this publication or parts thereof is permitted only under the provisions of the Copyright Law of the Publisher's location, in its current version, and permission for use must always be obtained from Springer. Permissions for use may be obtained through RightsLink at the Copyright Clearance Center. Violations are liable to prosecution under the respective Copyright Law.
The use of general descriptive names, registered names, trademarks, service marks, etc. in this publication does not imply, even in the absence of a specific statement, that such names are exempt from the relevant protective laws and regulations and therefore free for general use.
While the advice and information in this book are believed to be true and accurate at the date of publication, neither the authors nor the editors nor the publisher can accept any legal responsibility for any errors or omissions that may be made. The publisher makes no warranty, express or implied, with respect to the material contained herein.

Printed on acid-free paper

Springer is part of Springer Science+Business Media (www.springer.com)

Contents

1 **Geriatricians Involvement in Healthcare Changes** 1
James S. Powers

2 **Healthcare Changes and the Affordable Care Act: A Physician Call to Action Quality Improvement Organizations** 13
Adrienne D. Mims, Jane C. Pederson, and Jay A. Gold

3 **Leadership Opportunities for Physicians** 33
Laurie G. Jacobs

4 **The ABCs of ACOs** 65
Hope Glassberg, Anne Meara, Carolyn S. Blaum, and Laurie G. Jacobs

5 **Our Failing System: A Reasoned Approach Toward Single Payer** 83
Ed Weisbart

6 **Geriatric and Primary Care Workforce Development** 99
Michael R. Wasserman

7 **Medicare and Medicaid Coordination: Special Case of the Dual Eligible Beneficiary** 117
Gregg Warshaw and Peter A. DeGolia

8 **Care Management: From Channeling to Grace** 133
Michael R. Wasserman

9 **Program Evaluation: Defining and Measuring Appropriate Outcomes** 153
Peter A. Hollmann

10 **Targeting Interventions and Populations** 169
Adam G. Golden, Michael A. Silverman, and Thomas T.H. Wan

11 **Accountable Care Organizations: A Case Study in the Use of Care Coordination: Montefiore Medical Center** 187
    Hope Glassberg, Anne Meara, and Laurie G. Jacobs

12 **University of Michigan Case Study: The Physician Group Practice Demonstration** 199
    Caroline S. Blaum, Brent C. Williams, and David A. Spahlinger

Index 215

About the Editor

James S. Powers, M.D. received a B.A. cum laude from Wesleyan University (CT) in 1973 and M.D. with Distinction in Research from the University of Rochester (NY) in 1977 followed by residency in Internal Medicine at Cleveland Clinic and Case Western Reserve University Hospitals (1977–1980). He served in the USPHS National Health Service Corps (1980–1983) following which he was recruited to Vanderbilt to develop a Geriatric Medicine Program within the Division of General Internal Medicine. Dr. Powers is an Associate Professor of Medicine as well as Associate Professor of Gerontologic Nursing, Department of Family and Community Health. Author of over 90 papers, books, and book chapters, he has devoted his academic career to geriatric nutrition, education, and healthcare quality and safety. He has mentored over 1,700 trainees while at Vanderbilt and holds Fellowship in the American College of Physicians, American College of Nutrition, American Geriatrics Society, Gerontologic Society of America, and the Royal Society of Medicine. He serves as the Associate Clinical Director for the VA Tennessee Valley Geriatric Research Education and Clinical Center, and Program Director for the Vanderbilt Geriatric Fellowship. Dr. Powers' research interests include educational outcome evaluation, aging body composition, and models of geriatric care. He is PI of the Vanderbilt-Reynolds Geriatric Education Program, Co-PI of the Meharry Consortium Geriatric Education Center, and leads numerous clinical demonstration projects for the TVHS GRECC concerned with falls prevention, caregiver support, palliative care, treatment of agitated dementia, and health systems improvement.

Contributors and Biography

Contributors

Carolyn S. Blaum, M.D., M.S. Department of Medicine, Division of Geriatric Medicine and Palliative Care, NYU School of Medicine, NYU Langone Medical Center, New York, NY, USA

Peter A. DeGolia, M.D. Department of Family Medicine, University Hospitals Case Medical Center, Cleveland, OH, USA

Hope Glassberg, M.P.A. Care Management Organization, Montefiore Medical Center, Yonkers, NY, USA

Jay A. Gold, M.D., J.D., M.P.H. MetaStar, Inc, Madison, WI, USA

Adam G. Golden, M.D., M.B.A. Department of Internal Medicine, University of Central Florida College of Medicine, Orlando VA Medical Center, Orlando, FL, USA

Peter A. Hollmann, M.D. Division of Geriatrics, Blue Cross & Blue Shield of RI, Providence, RI, USA

Laurie G. Jacobs, M.D. Department of Medicine, Montefiore Medical Center and Albert Einstein College of Medicine, Bronx, NY, USA

Anne Meara, BSN, M.B.A. Care Management Organization, Montefiore Medical Center, Yonkers, NY, USA

Adrienne D. Mims, M.D., M.P.H. Medicare Quality Improvement, Quality Improvement Organization, Alliant GMCF, Atlanta, GA, USA

American Health Quality Association, Washington, DC, USA

Jane C. Pederson, M.D., M.S. Medical Affairs, Stratis Health, Bloomington, MN, USA

James S. Powers, M.D. Department of Medicine, Vanderbilt University School of Medicine, Tennessee Valley Geriatric Research, Education, and Clinical Center, Nashville, TN, USA

Michael A. Silverman, M.D., M.P.H. Geriatrics & Extended Care, West Palm Beach Veterans Affairs Medical Center, Riviera Beach, FL, USA

David A. Spahlinger, M.D. Internal Medicine, University of Michigan, Ann Arbor, MI, USA

Thomas T.H. Wan, Ph.D. College of Health and Public Affairs, University of Central Florida, Orlando, FL, USA

Gregg Warshaw, M.D. Geriatric Medicine Program and Department of Family and Community Medicine, College of Medicine, University of Cincinnati, Cincinnati, OH, USA

Michael R. Wasserman, M.D. Division of Geriatric Medicine, University of Colorado Denver, Woodland Hills, CA, USA

Ed Weisbart, M.D. Internal Medicine, Barnes Jewish Medical Center, Creve Coeur, MO, USA

Brent C. Williams, M.D., M.P.H. Internal Medicine, University of Michigan, Ann Arbor, MI, USA

Biography

Caroline S. Blaum, M.D., M.S. is Professor of Geriatric Medicine and the Director of the Division of Geriatric Medicine and Palliative Care at the New York University Langone Medical Center. Dr. Blaum served as the Assistant Dean for Clinical Affairs and Associate Medical Director of the University of Michigan's Faculty Group Practice, directing the UM Health System's Population Health Program. From 2005 to 2010 she led the University of Michigan's efforts in the Medicare Physician Group Practice Demonstration. She is the American Geriatrics Society's representative to the AMA Physician Consortium for Performance Improvement and sits on its Executive Committee. She currently is Chair of the NIH Aging Systems and Geriatrics Study Section. She has a geriatrics practice at NYULMC and consults on older adult patients in the acute hospital. She is very active in teaching internal medicine and geriatrics to medical students, house officers and geriatrics fellows.

Peter DeGolia, M.D. is a Professor of Family Medicine and Community Health at Case Western Reserve University School of Medicine. He works as a geriatrician and hospice/palliative medicine physician at University Hospitals Case Medical Center. He is the Medical Director of the McGregor PACE program in Cleveland, Ohio.

Hope Glassberg, M.P.A. is the Director of Public Policy for Montefiore Medical Center. She provides policy analysis and strategic planning support related to the accountable care initiatives of the Montefiore Care Management Organization, providing the management services infrastructure for Montefiore's integrated provider association. Previously, she served as the Special Assistant to the Director of the Center for Medicaid and CHIP Services at the US Department of Health and Human Services in Washington DC. She also worked as a Policy Analyst at the Council of State Governments Justice Center, a criminal justice policy non-profit, and as a reporter and freelance writer for publications including *Dow Jones Newswires, The Wall Street Journal,* and the *New York Times*.

Jay A. Gold, M.D., J.D., M.P.H. is Senior Vice President and Chief Medical Officer of MetaStar, Madison, WI. Te is founding chair of the Physician Leadership Network of the American Health Quality Association. He is a certified specialist in preventive medicine and public health and in legal medicine. He holds a law degree from New York University and an MPH from Harvard University. He currently serves on the faculties of the Medical College of Wisconsin, the University of Wisconsin School of Medicine and Public Health, and Marquette University Law School. Dr. Gold serves on the Executive Committee of the AMA Physician Consortium for Performance Improvement, and on the Board of Directors of the Wisconsin Medical Society. He has chaired the Wisconsin Heart Disease and Stroke Alliance and the Wisconsin Independent Review Board. He has published and lectured extensively on the subjects of health care quality, law, policy, and ethics.

Adam G. Golden, M.D. is an Associate Professor of Medicine at the University of Central Florida College of Medicine, Department of Internal Medicine, Orlando, FL. He is also the Associate Chief of Staff for Geriatrics and Extended Care at the Orlando Veterans Affairs Medical Center.

Peter Hollmann, M.D. is an Assistant Clinical Professor of Medicine at Warren Alpert School of Medicine, Brown University, where he received his graduate and post-graduate education in Internal Medicine and Geriatrics. He practices primary care geriatrics and is Associate Chief Medical Officer of Blue Cross and Blue Shield in RI. He was a leader in the American Geriatrics Society's work in shaping the ACA and has helped in creating performance measures for geriatrics as a member of the NCQA Geriatrics Measures Advisory Panel. His current focus is on practice transformation in RI as chairman of the data and evaluation committee of a multi-payer PCMH demonstration program.

Laurie G. Jacobs, M.D. is Vice Chairman for Clinical and Educational Programs for the Department of Medicine at Montefiore Medical Center and Albert Einstein College of Medicine. She is responsible for program development; physician recruitment, productivity, compensation, and credentialing; and oversight of training programs, for more than 1,000 physicians in general, hospital and specialty internal medicine. She represents the Department for all Montefiore Medical Center and Montefiore Health System endeavors and serves as a board member of their Pioneer ACO, the Bronx Accountable Care Network. In addition, she is Professor of Medicine, in the Division of Geriatrics, having previously served as the Geriatrics Division Chief. She continues to practice and teach geriatrics in addition to her leadership roles.

Anne Meara, BSN, M.B.A. is the Associate Vice President of Network Care Management at Montefiore. She has responsibilities both within Montefiore's delivery system and at CMO, Montefiore Care Management. At Montefiore she has implemented a comprehensive care management program that incorporates intensive medical and behavioral case management, chronic care management, and care transitions programs that involve over 500 staff across the continuum of care. Montefiore is 1 of 32 Pioneer ACOs. She also has responsibility for implementing and overseeing all aspects of care management activities associated with the Pioneer ACO.

Adrienne Mims, M.D., M.P.H. is a board-certified family medicine/geriatrician with over 30 years of primary care, consultative, and home care geriatric experience. Dr. Mims has worked as a medical administrator for 25 years in the fields of quality measurement, quality improvement, health care systems re-design, patient education, preventive health, and population research. In her current role, she serves as Vice President, Chief Medical Officer at the Georgia Quality Improvement Organization, where she has been since 2009. She serves on the Board of Directors for the American Geriatric Society as a member of the AMA Physician Consortium for Performance Improvement QI Committee and as a member of the NCQA Geriatric Measurement Advisory Panel.

Jane C. Pederson, M.D., M.S. practices in the long-term care setting and has served as nursing home medical director. In her role at Stratis Health, she provides leadership and clinical guidance to health care quality and safety initiatives. Dr. Pederson is board certified in internal medicine and geriatrics. She is an active member of a number of state and national health care organizations and participates in various work groups that focus on topics relevant to older individuals. She received her M.D. and completed her residency at the University of Minnesota. In addition, she holds an M.S. in Health Services Research and Policy also from the University of Minnesota.

James S. Powers, M.D. is Associate Professor of Medicine at Vanderbilt University School of Medicine and Associate Clinical Director at the Tennessee Valley Healthcare System, Geriatrics Research Education and Clinical Center, Nashville, TN. He is the Geriatrics Fellowship Program Director, and for over three decades has developed geriatric healthcare models and educational programs throughout Middle Tennessee. He focuses on evaluating educational and clinical outcomes, maintains a large practice, and teaches geriatrics to healthcare professionals of all disciplines. For his work, he was awarded the Marsha Goodwin-Beck VA Interdisciplinary Award for Excellence in Geriatric Clinical Care Delivery. Dr. Powers chaired two national symposia on physician involvement in healthcare changes for the American Geriatrics Society in 2012 and 2013. This work grew out of that collaboration.

Michael A. Silverman, M.D. is the Associate Chief of Geriatrics and Extended Care at the West Palm Beach Veterans Affairs Medical Center and a Professor of Medicine (voluntary) at the University of Miami Miller School of Medicine.

David A. Spahlinger, M.D. serves as the Senior Associate Dean for Clinical Affairs in the University of Michigan Medical School and as the Executive Director of the University of Michigan's physician group, the Faculty Group Practice. In 2004, the Faculty Group Practice board of directors applied for the Centers of Medicaid and Medicare Physician Group Practice Demonstration Project. The University of Michigan's Faculty Group Practice saved money for Medicare in each of the 5 years. Dr. Spahlinger is past chair of the AAMC Advisory Committee for Healthcare and past chair of the AAMC Group on Faculty Practice. Dr. Spahlinger is a hospitalist and still attends on the inpatient wards.

Thomas T.H. Wan, Ph.D., M.H.S. is a Professor of the Doctoral program and the Associate Dean of Research in the College of Health and Public Affairs, University of Central Florida.

Gregg Warshaw, M.D. is a Professor of Family Medicine and Community Medicine, Director of the Geriatric Medicine Program, and the Martha Betty Semmons Professor of Geriatric Medicine, at the University of Cincinnati, in Ohio. He is a 2013–2014 Atlantic Philanthropies Health and Aging Policy fellow.

Michael Wasserman, M.D. has practiced primary care and consultative geriatrics for over two decades, beginning at Kaiser Permanente, where he first developed a geriatric consult clinic. He then developed and led GeriMed of America, as president of a physician practice management company that operated senior health clinics. Finally, he co-found Senior Care of Colorado, with Dr. Don Murphy. Over this period he has interviewed and hired scores of geriatricians, nurse practitioners, and physician assistants in order to provide primary care to older adults. He continues to consult widely, teach, and contributes his keen insight to national geriatrics societies.

Ed Weisbart, M.D. chairs the Missouri chapter of Physicians for a National Health Program, part of the 26-year-old 18,000 member non-profit organization that advocates for improving Medicare and providing it to all Americans. He also volunteers as a physician in a variety of safety net clinics and other non-profits across the St. Louis area. He practiced family medicine at Rush Medical Center in Chicago for 20 years before moving to St. Louis in 2003 to become chief medical officer at Express Scripts. He retired from that position in 2010 and now devotes most of his time to advocating for social justice in healthcare. He is an Assistant Professor of Clinical Medicine at Washington University in St. Louis. He has had several articles published in national medical journals regarding the healthcare needs of the uninsured. The St. Louis Post Dispatch and other local media have printed several of his op-eds about single payer healthcare and Medicaid expansion. He was recognized by the Academy of Managed Care Pharmacy with their Grassroots Advocacy Award.

Brent Williams, M.D., M.P.H. is Associate Professor of Medicine at the University of Michigan (UM), currently serves as Medical Director of the UM Complex Care

Management program where he has developed clinical programs to improve care and decrease inappropriate health care expenses among high-utilizing patients with combined medical, mental health, substance abuse disorders, and/or poverty and homelessness. He has focused on medical education, faculty development, and development of new models of clinical practice for vulnerable populations. An active primary care physician for over 25 years, he has authored over 50 publications and served as chief editor for the 2013 book *Hospitalists' Guide to the Care of Older Patients*.

Introduction

Physician Involvement in Healthcare Reform

Background Information

For over 100 years, six US presidents have tried and the Obama Administration succeeded in changing the fundamental rules of the American Healthcare System to improve access to affordable healthcare. From 2014 to 2023 we will spend $180 billion yearly to increase access, realign incentives, create new partnerships, scale new models of care, and develop outcome measures [1].

The Affordable Care Act (ACA) of 2010 established a Centers for Medicare and Medicaid Services (CMS) Center for Innovation evaluating over 4,000 demonstration pilots of new models of care, from patient centered medical homes, transition of care continuums, prescribing safety projects, collaborative care models, and accountable care organizations.

From a physician's perspective, The ACA does several important things. It (1) establishes healthcare as a requirement, (2) promotes the health of patients, (3) removes barriers to providing healthcare by providing access, (4) emphasizes primary care, and (5) incentivizes physicians to improve quality and slow the rate of cost growth. This is a special time in healthcare, and physicians can honestly ask "Where do I fit in?" Indeed, this is an opportunity to provide leadership.

Geriatricians care for the sickest and most costly segment of the population. CMS estimates that this 10 % of the population accounts for over 70 % of healthcare costs. We need geriatrics involvement as innovators for new models of care and to ensure that work flow, clinician acceptability, and patient-centeredness is preserved. This book will serve to provide guidance, examples, and information on processes and timelines for physicians.

There is much to learn about. Many elements of the ACA are yet to be implemented. There are many healthcare decisions to be made. There will be many new models of care to evaluate and expand. We need dedicated, informed, and energetic physician leaders committed to providing the best healthcare to all our citizens. I hope you will accept the challenge.

James S. Powers, M.D.
Department of Medicine,
Vanderbilt University School of Medicine,
Tennessee Valley Geriatric Research,
Education, and Clinical Center,
Nashville, TN, USA

Reference

1. Congressional Budget Office. Gross cost for ACA coverage provisions. Retrieved from http://www.cbo.gov/publication/44176

Chapter 1
Geriatricians Involvement in Healthcare Changes

James S. Powers

Introduction

Physicians have traditionally strived to improve healthcare quality and continually develop new models of care. As innovators and leaders in the provision of healthcare, it is imperative that they understand the complex relationships between quality, efficiency, and value which are driving US healthcare changes in an unprecedented manner. The continuing rise in cost of US healthcare is unsustainable, making price and quality transparency the new rules of engagement.

Geographic variations in spending, healthcare access, and population health outcomes all reflect decisions contributed at least in part, by physicians. Physicians understand what is best for the patient and are aware of clinical realities. Healthcare system shifts from producer-driven to patient-centered outcome drivers demand physician involvement, and the time is now.

The Affordable Care Act has created a critical opportunity to contribute to increasing the value of healthcare services to all citizens. It is appropriate that physicians be among the leaders in promoting models of care. Geriatricians, especially, care for the sickest, most vulnerable, and most costly of the population. Geriatrician-led models are the historic innovations of many care processes shown to improve care. This is extremely relevant to healthcare changes. Geriatricians have a vast knowledge about caring for older people. They also have demonstrated an extraordinary and sustained commitment to improving the quality of life for older people. This value-added input is not clearly recognized by physician peers or healthcare organizations.

J.S. Powers, M.D. (✉)
Department of Medicine, Vanderbilt University School of Medicine,
Tennessee Valley Geriatric Research, Education, and Clinical Center,
7159 Vanderbilt Medical Center East, Nashville, TN 37232, USA
e-mail: james.powers@vanderbilt.edu

Geriatric models of care include many approaches to care that are proven to be more effective, when appropriately targeted and applied, in treating older people. These include access, design, and outcome assessments in primary care settings, disease state management, hospital and post-acute care settings. These models demonstrate maintenance of function, cost avoidance, and reduced complications for selected frail elderly populations. They provide solutions benefitting older adults in proven and cost-effective ways that enhance quality throughout the healthcare system.

Acute Care for Elderly (ACE) Units provide interdisciplinary care, comprehensive review, and an environment of care conducive to early rehabilitation and patient-centered care, improving function and reducing iatrogenic and hospital acquired conditions [1]. These geriatric laboratories, present since the 1970s remain few in number nationally.

Geriatric Resources for Assessing Care for Elders (GRACE) team care, is a recent cost-effective team care model that improves the health of frail older adults by working with patients in their homes and communities to manage health problems, track changing care needs, and leverage social services. In the GRACE model, interdisciplinary teams guided by care protocols, improve outcomes. Increases in preventive and chronic care are offset by reduced acute care costs [2].

The Program for All-inclusive Care for Elderly (PACE) provides integrated acute medical care and long term care services to frail seniors. PACE provides a community-based alternative to nursing home care when nursing home placement seems necessary. PACE uses blended Medicare and Medicaid financing to provide care, and reduces mortality and improves function [3]. Present since the 1970s, the costs of PACE home based long term care are offset by avoidance of nursing home costs.

Assessing Care of Vulnerable Elders (ACOVE) is a series of evidence-based best practices for 26 conditions affecting frail elders [4] developed by collaboration between the American Geriatrics Society and the Rand Corporation. ACOVE addresses promotion of hospital safety for vulnerable elders, reducing hospital acquired conditions, IDT (interdisciplinary team) care, assessment of delirium in hospitalized patients, setting patient-specific goals for blood pressure (avoiding hypotension) and identifying and addressing risk factors for falls and decubiti.

Additional disease state innovations include development of best practices for medication safety and identifying potentially inappropriate medications (PIMS) [5], best practice recommendations for diabetes management [6], especially documenting the risks of hypoglycemia, and developing a clinical algorithm for patients with multiple co-morbidities [7].

Transitions of care programs for home care following hospitalization utilizing advance practice nurse-directed discharge planning and follow-up protocols have shown promise in reducing early repeat hospitalizations [8]. Similarly, the Coleman Care Transitions Program, a patient-centered self-management program coordinated by a health coach, has also reduced repeat hospitalizations [9]. INTERACT is a nursing home quality improvement intervention providing tools and strategies to assist nursing home staff in the early identification, assessment, and communication regarding changes in resident status [10]. The improved communication and hand-offs between hospital and nursing home, appears to prevent avoidable rehospitalizations. These innovative ideas are the basis of many of the new models of care encouraged by CMS and are centered around patient-specific goals, quality, and safety, reflecting cost avoidance on other components of the healthcare system.

Nurses Improving the Care of HealthSystem Elders (NICHE) is dedicated to the principle that all older adults be given sensitive and exemplary care. The program began in 1981 and is now operating in 450 US hospitals. NICHE helps participating hospitals build nursing leadership capabilities to enact system-level changes targeting the unique needs of older adults and put evidence-based knowledge into practice. NICHE tools exert important influences over care provided to older adult patients by increasing the organizational support for geriatric nursing [11].

A hospital at home (admission avoidance) program seeks to provide hospital-level care for selected patients in the patient's home. Operating as an enhanced interdisciplinary team home-care program, this model shows promise of achieving hospital quality standards with shorter lengths of stay. There are also suggestions of reduced complications in addition to increased family and patient satisfaction [12].

What Is Driving Healthcare Changes?

Healthcare absorbs an increasing proportion of government and private sector spending without proportional benefits healthcare status and outcomes. According to the Budget of the US Government, healthcare equates to approximately 19 % of overall spending, exceeding both education and defense spending. Yet the US spends more per capita on healthcare than any other nation, including a 70 % increase in per-beneficiary Medicare spending between 2000 and 2012 and total healthcare expenditures continue to rise (Fig. 1.1). At the same time the US falls at

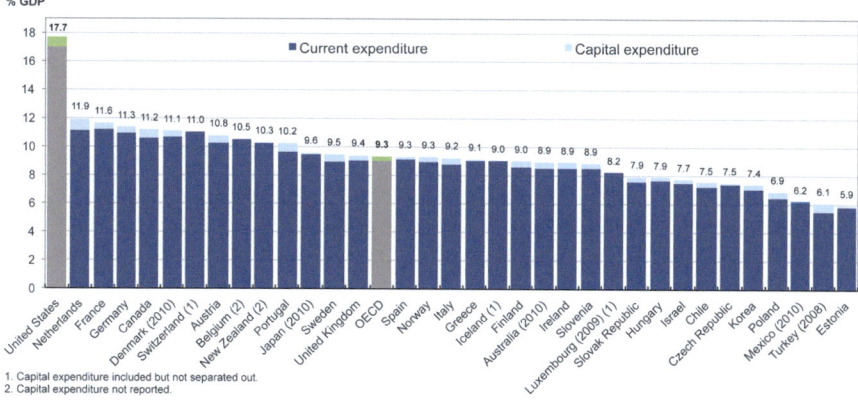

Fig. 1.1 Total health expenditure per capita, $US PPP (OECD (2013), *OECD Health Statistics 2013*, OECD Publishing, Paris. http://dx.doi.org/10.1787/health-data-en)

37 overall for health outcomes, trailing many nations in infant mortality, life expectancy, patient safety, healthcare access, disease management and measures of health disparities [13].

Healthcare costs have risen at an unsustainable rate, and there are serious mismatches between cost, outcomes, and distribution of health resources in the US. This curious combination of high cost and poor outcomes has engendered much criticism and concern for inefficiency, waste, and profiteering incentivized by a fee for service and procedure-based reimbursement system. Major changes in healthcare financing and delivery are inevitable, with an emphasis on reducing overhead expenses and costs associated with little or no outcome benefit. The message is clear, the time is now for physicians to engage in the process of change, not stubbornly grasping at long-standing silos of specialty care, but real involvement to create a seamless flow of coordinated care – at the starting gate.

Physicians control 80 % of healthcare spending, including the location where patients are seen, laboratory and diagnostic testing, and treatment and further referrals. While physicians are not the only ones responsible for controlling healthcare costs, real cost containment requires that all relevant stakeholders are mobilized to ensure that patient centered care is at the core of any changes. Physicians cannot be absent, indeed they must lead these changes. As collaborators and innovators, geriatricians are a natural force in leading healthcare change. Indeed all physicians now have a unique opportunity to serve as leaders. Furthermore, because of their credibility, the population looks to them for direction in healthcare matters.

The triple aim of the Institute for Healthcare Improvement is to improve the patient's experience of care, improve the health of the population, and reduce the per-capita cost of health care. This focus on quality, efficiency, and value is forcing health systems to pay attention to older, vulnerable patients because they consume disproportionate resources. The Agency for Healthcare Research and Quality [14] reported that approximately 50 % of US healthcare expenditures are attributed to 5 % of patients [14]. CMS estimates that 70 % healthcare costs are related to chronic illness, and the Medicare population utilizes 32 % of resources in the last 2 months of life. In 2009 the Medical Expenditure Panel survey found that the sickest 10 % of patients accounted for 65 % of all healthcare expenses in the United States. Moreover, there is great disparity in healthcare outcomes that is not explained by cost. Geographic variation in healthcare costs in the Medicare fee for service population has fueled the perception of an inefficient US healthcare system which lacks transparency (Fig. 1.2). Elucidating the causes of geographic variation and comparing the effects of new models of care on usual costs and processes of care are important priorities for comparative effectiveness research. An Institute of medicine report suggests that 73 % of the variation is in post-acute care and 27 % inpatient care [15]. The reality of mal-distribution of resources, cost, quality, and outcomes his driving process standardization, more organized and coordinated systems focusing on cost consciousness in medical decisions, as well as greater price and quality transparency.

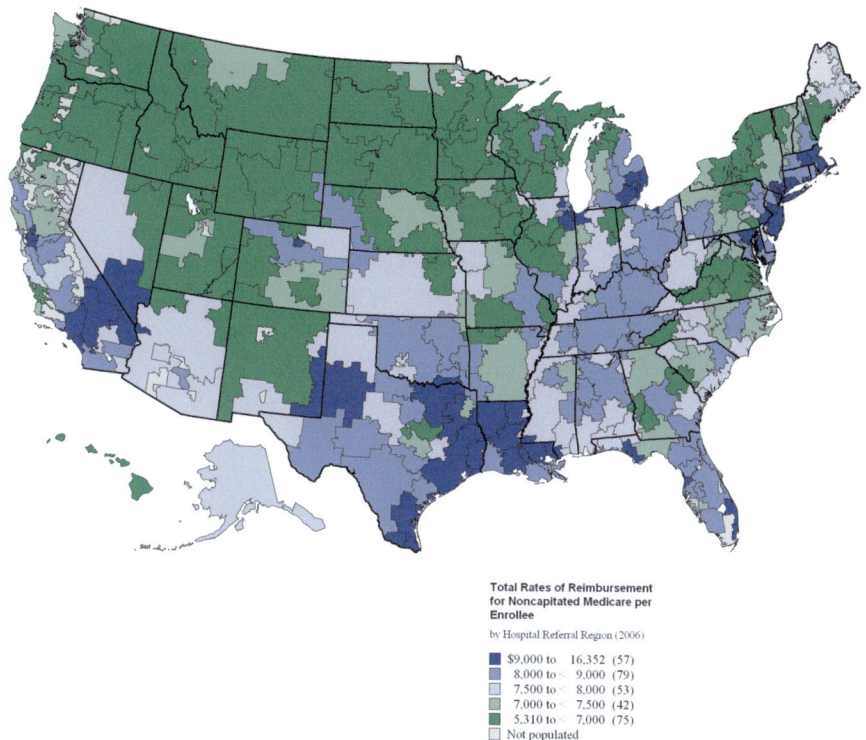

Fig. 1.2 National variation in medicare spending (Fisher ES, Goodman DC, Skinner JS, Bronner KK. Health care spending, quality and outcomes. Hanover, NH: Trustees of Dartmouth College, February 27, 2009. http://www.dartmouthatlas.org/downloads/reports/Spending_Brief_022709.pdf)

Globally the population of older people is growing rapidly. According to the UN World Population Prospectus, the US population over age 65, currently at 13 %, will make up 20 % of the population by 2040 and is projected to stabilize thereafter (Fig. 1.3). Due to these population dynamics, support for Medicare and Social Security rests on fewer taxpayers. Currently there are 2.9 workers per retiree and this is ratio is projected to be 2:1 in 2030, with future projections falling to 1:1 making the current structure financially unsustainable. Medicare Trust Fund, which covers hospitalization, will begin to decline by 2018 with depletion by 2026 according to the latest trustee report (Fig. 1.4). These realities are forcing a reassessment of the US healthcare system and are major drivers of the Affordable Care Act of 2010.

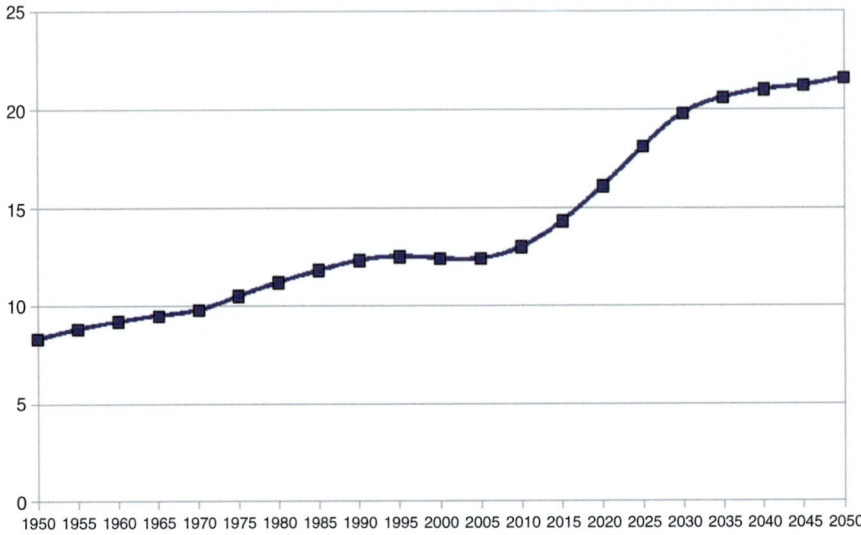

Fig. 1.3 Percentage of US population over age 65, 1950-2052 (Source: UN World Population Prospectus 2008. *Creative Common Attribution 3.0 Unported License*)

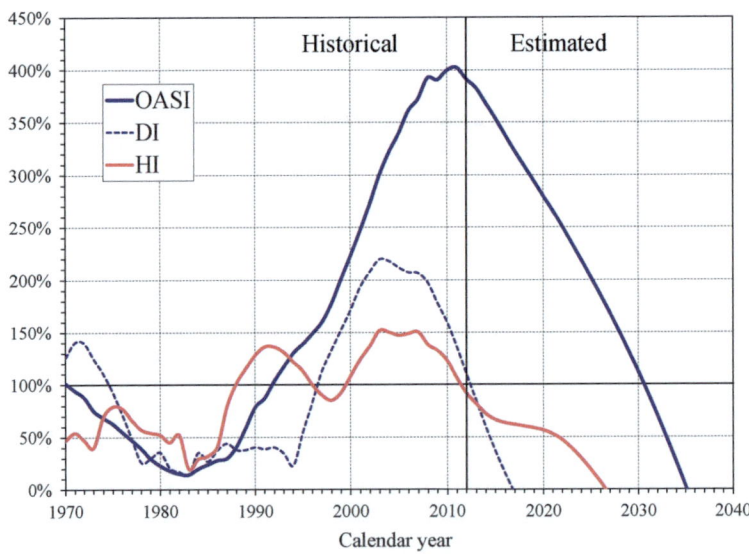

Fig. 1.4 OASI (Social Security), DI, (Disability) and HI (Medicare) Trust Fund Ratios [*Asset reserves as a percentage of annual cost*] (http://www.ssa.gov/oact/trsum/. Accessed 22 Apr 2014)

Healthcare Innovation

There are several ways to address increased costs to Medicare from this growing elderly population: cost controls, reduced benefits, or increased premiums. Naturally, neither of these approaches has any political momentum. Raising the eligibility age, increasing the payroll tax, or tying benefits to income level all adversely affect different segments of the population. There is therefore a major focus on controlling costs and improving efficiency. The US has about a 10 year window to reign-in runaway costs through improved care delivery, elimination of waste, and improved healthcare outcomes, and expanding access to preventive and primary care. Value-based purchasing, tying provider reimbursement to outcomes representing real value to patients, is a powerful new force designed to change provider incentives and leverage the healthcare delivery system to sustain change over time. This change in incentives will require widespread adoption by all payers and utilization of quality improvement teams in all healthcare settings. Performance on outcomes measures may negatively impact hospitals that care for more disadvantaged patients.

New models of care with varying degrees of risk will be required for individual and provider organizations to take advantage of these incentives. Many of these have shown promise, but have not been widely disseminated. The Patient Centered Medical Home involves team-based patient-centered primary care and disease management and is low risk. It may reduce return visits and achieve higher rates of disease management goals, and has been used most widely for five million patients in the Veterans' Administration [16]. Transitions of care programs reduce re-hospitalization among targeted populations by up to 50 % [8] and utilize care management teams to improve communication and patient education, as well as enhanced follow-up.

Hospital safety programs for specific conditions strive to reduce hospital acquired conditions among vulnerable populations. These programs are promoted by CMS's Partnership for Patients, part of the Tenth Scope of Work of the state Quality Improvement Organizations (QIO). State QIO's work under contract with CMS to assist physician offices, hospitals, nursing homes, home health agencies, and community partners to align care processes with national standards to ensure quality of care of beneficiaries. Among the hospital safety programs are ten priority areas (Table 1.1).

Table 1.1 Hospital acquired conditions: ten priority areas of focus	
	1. Adverse drug events
	2. Catheter-associated urinary tract infections
	3. Central line associated blood stream infections
	4. Injuries from falls and immobility
	5. Obstetrical adverse events
	6. Pressure ulcers
	7. Surgical site infections
	8. Venous thromboembolism
	9. Ventilator-associated pneumonia
	10. Reducing readmissions

While integrated delivery systems of the 1990s failed to control costs, accountable care organizations (ACO's) including variable risk strategies, hold a promise of cost avoidance, maintenance of quality, and improved population health. ACO's are formed by voluntary healthcare organization providers and suppliers of services who accept blocks of unselected fee for service Medicare patients provided by CMS. These partners accept shared responsibility to coordinate care and deliver seemless, high quality care. Payment is dependent on the assumed risk structure and outcomes connected to coordination of care, disease management, and transitions of care. Reimbursement is thus linked to processes rather than production metrics. This is in stark contrast to fragmented care where providers receive different, disconnected payments. Early reports on the Pioneer ACO's, showed that 27 of the 35 exceeded fiscal targets [17].

There is early evidence that the wider community of physicians may be initially hesitant to lead and adopt new models of care which include more cost and value consciousness in medical decisions. These include bundled payments and team-based care strategies, decreased disparity in reimbursement among specialties, and changing incentives from fee for service models in favor of performance payment with shared risk [18]. This is indeed unfortunate as the healthcare system shifts from producer-driven to outcome (patient-centered) drivers with mandated reporting of individual quality measures. We urgently need physician input accepting key roles in making important decisions. There is tremendous opportunity for younger physicians especially to step-up and lead the way. Physicians understand what is best for the patient and are aware of clinical realities. They can work to ensure optimum patient care and physician acceptability, and enhance quality [19]. Physicians and their respective medical societies will need to guide consensus building efforts to develop patient centered quality and outcome measures targeting the things that matter, i.e. accurate and timely diagnoses, judicious testing, appropriate treatment interventions, and caring for the increasing numbers of patients with multiple co-morbidities and functional limitations. These measures must support patient valued physician characteristics including empathy, honesty, respect, and thoroughness. If they do not accept this challenge, physicians risk marginalization and all of society suffers.

Many professional societies have followed the lead of the American College of Physicians' Choosing Wisely Campaign, developing high value care recommendations. These are specialty-specific guidelines for cost-conscious care which eliminates unsafe and low value services that generate expenses with potential harm or no benefit. Only time will tell if new incentives and models of care and physician involvement, sustained over time, will be effective in improving the US healthcare system.

Leadership Is a function of (Expertise, Change, Risk, Persistence, and Trust)

A wise man once said: "If people follow you, you're a leader." Physicians have great potential when they become involved as agents of change. Viewed as experts in healthcare matters, the public has a high regard for physicians and in fact looks to them for direction and leadership in matters involving health. In my experience, the public, government, and business as a rule, still defers to physicians as the healthcare experts. This acknowledgement is not only regarding personal health, but also in policy arenas. Physician organizations are especially urged to provide input, helping to shape critical healthcare decisions.

Leadership can take many forms, but it is always personalized. And it is always about change. There is always one person, a leader, who begins anything. A leader possesses competency and engenders trust to create a shared context, inspiring others to work together to achieve common goals. This creates a structured support to guide transformation. Leadership involves risk tolerance, yes and persistence. A leader is motivated and passionate and ignites this in others. Some leaders lead by example and followers respond by imitation. Others facilitate shared leadership functions and provide advice to influence and enable changes at all levels.

Although many seek leadership positions in order to influence change, in truth leadership occurs at many levels and different types of leadership require different skill sets. Some leaders create a membership-participatory organization style rather than a top-down environment. These leaders contribute experience to influence decision making and are foundational for building a culture of quality and safety [20]. Their influence is critical in creating measurable objectives and work plans leading to system-wide changes. They may initiate activities voluntarily and function in acting roles, creating new positions for others. Informal leadership roles do not always provide official recognition, so these agents of change often possess a selfless dedication. But all are leaders.

Leaders have a clear vision with a discipline and commitment to work for change. They frame the issues and give a sense of scale, engaging others in causes bigger than themselves. Authentic leaders are competent and personally trustworthy. They are good communicators, building relationships through empathy, understanding, and inspiration. An inclusive leadership style acknowledges other's values and points of view, and energizes them to create committed action. While the mind weighs facts, the heart seeks meaning, and the effective leader manages both to give meaning and relevance to the cause for change.

Many true leaders are conferred leaders, acknowledged either formally or informally for their competence and experience and consulted for their expertise to guide the discussion, formally and informally. They stimulate and support the planning, implementation, and evaluation of change processes. These agents of change form a foundation for building a culture of quality and safety, complementing existing organizational structures. A responsible organization ignores sound advice at its own peril. Many physicians adopt executive and administrative responsibilities, but may not be recognized as executives. Not all leaders are in charge of institutional levers, nor appointed by others in authority. Indeed, appointment to positions of authority can potentially alter a leaders' commitment to change, placing them in conflict with new and different priorities. Witness the fate of many politicians elected to office with promises of change only to be confronted with the realities of competing demands of the office. Regrettably, some individuals appointed to positions of authority are not, in fact, effective leaders.

Becoming involved as physician leaders includes volunteering to quality improvement and safety committees. It involves accepting appointments to hospital, organization, and practice boards. Familiarity with organizational performance metrics and outcomes measures are also critical prerequisites to articulating strategies to move organizations.

Barriers to Change

Many good ideas are not always followed. But the specter of Medicare insolvency and the continued rise of US healthcare spending is forcing us to focus on increased costs. There are many good proposals: shared resources, improved communication, incentivizing shared outcomes. Visibility is a potential problem to an evolving leader. Marketing, consultation, and being helpful to organizations are effective strategies for the spokesperson advocating change. It's all about achieving common overlapping goals, a win-win-win, and being helpful as well as adaptable. It's not about who gets credit. In the final analysis, it's the outcome – not who's the genius behind the idea.

Resistance to change is expected from those enjoying the benefits of current fee for service, procedural, and volume-based system. Rallying under the banner of choice, freedom to select providers becomes a false promise for disenfranchised populations when access is denied, care delayed, and preventive services nonexistent. It also takes leadership to address the health needs of vulnerable populations, as these do not traditionally participate in the decision making process for benefits, and are not prone to self-management.

Incentives must be changed to enhance collaboration. It would be unfortunate if the healthcare system has to fail, the public has to suffer more, spend more before healthcare changes. There are many new models of care to provide guidance and incentivize change.

The next decade will require an all-hands-on-deck approach to participate in meaningful, effective, patient-centered, and physician- directed change.

References

1. Fox MT, Sidani S, Persaud M, Tregunno D, Maimets I, Brooks D, O'Brien K. Acute care for elders components of acute geriatric unit care: systematic descriptive review. J Am Geriatr Soc. 2013;61:939–46.
2. Counsell SR, Callahan CM, Tu W, Stump TE, Arling GW. Cost analysis of the geriatric resources for assessment and care of elders care management intervention. J Am Geriatr Soc. 2009;57:1420–6.
3. http://www.npaonline.org/website/download.asp?id=2030&title=PACE:__An_Evaluation_-_2005. Accessed 22 April 2014.
4. ACOVE. Measuring medical care provided to vulnerable elders: the assessing care of vulnerable elders-3 (ACOVE-3) quality indicators. J Am Geriatr Soc 2007;55(S-2):S-247–487.
5. American Geriatrics Society 2012 Beers Criteria Expert Panel. American Geriatrics Society updated Beers criteria for potentially inappropriate medication use in older adults. J Am Geriatr Soc. 2012;60:616–31.
6. Kirkman MS, Jones Briscoe V, Clark N, et al. Diabetes in older adults: a consensus report. J Am Geriatr Soc. 2012;60:2342–56.
7. American Geriatrics Society Expert Panel on the Care of Older Adults with Multimorbidity. Patient-centered care for older adults with multiple chronic conditions: a stepwise approach. J Am Geriatr Soc. 2012;60:E1–25.
8. Naylor MD, Brooten DA, Campbell RL, Maislin G, McCauley KM, Schwartz JS. Transitional care of older adults hospitalized with heart failure: a randomized, controlled trial. J Am Geriatr Soc. 2004;52:675–84.
9. Ouslander J, Lamb G, Tappan R, et al. Interventions to reduce hospitalizations from nursing homes: evaluation of the INTERACT II collaborative quality improvement project. J Am Geriatr Soc. 2011;59:745–53.
10. Coleman EA, Smith JD, Frank JC, Min S, Parry C, Kramer AM. Preparing patients and caregivers to participate in care delivered across settings: the care transitions intervention. J Am Geriatr Soc. 2004;42:1817–25.
11. Boltz M, Capezuti E, Bowar-Ferres S, et al. Changes in the geriatric care environment associated with NICHE (Nurses Improving Care for Health System Elders). Geriatr Nurs. 2008;29:176–85.
12. Leff B, Burton L, Mader SL, et al. Hospital at home: feasibility and outcomes of a program to provide hospital-level care at home for acutely ill older patients. Ann Intern Med. 2005;143:798–808.
13. World Health Organization. The world health report 2000 – health systems: improving performance. Geneva: World Health Organization; 2000.
14. Cohen SB, Yu W. The concentration and persistence in the level of health expenditures over time: estimates for the U.S. population, 2008–2009. Statistical brief #354. Rockville: The Agency for Healthcare Research and Quality; 2012. http://meps.ahrq.gov/mepsweb/data_files/publications/st354/stat354.shtml.
15. Institute of Medicine. Interim report of the committee on geographic variation in health care spending and promotion of high value care: preliminary committee observations. 2014. http://books.nap.edu/openbook.php?record_id=18308. Accessed 22 April 2014.
16. Rosland AM, Nelson K, Sun H, et al. The patient-centered medical home in the Veterans Health Administration. Am J Manag Care. 2013;19:e-263–72.
17. http://www.brookings.edu/research/opinions/2013/07/25-assessing-pioneer-acos-patel.
18. Tilburt JC, Wynia MK, Sheeler RD, et al. Views of US physicians about controlling health care costs. JAMA. 2013;310:380–8.
19. Goodall A. Physician-leaders and hospital performance: is there an association? Soc Sci Med. 2011;73:535–9.
20. Trastek VF, Neil W, Hamilton JD, Niles E. Leadership models in health care – a case for servant leadership. Mayo Clin Proc. 2014;89:374–81.

Chapter 2
Healthcare Changes and the Affordable Care Act: A Physician Call to Action Quality Improvement Organizations

Adrienne D. Mims, Jane C. Pederson, and Jay A. Gold

Abbreviations

AAA	Area Agency on Aging
AAFP	American Academy of Family Physicians
AARP	American Association of Retired Persons
AGS	American Geriatric Society

Disclaimer The analyses upon which this publication is based were performed under Contract Number HHSM-500-2011-GA10C, entitled CMS10thSOW sponsored by the Centers for Medicare and Medicaid Services, Department of Health and Human Services. The content of this publication does not necessarily reflect the views or policies of the Department of Health and Human Services, nor does mention of trade names, commercial products, or organizations imply endorsement by the U.S. Government.

The authors assume full responsibility for the accuracy and completeness of the ideas presented. This article is a direct result of the Health Care Quality Improvement Program initiated by the Centers for Medicare and Medicaid Services, which has encouraged identification of quality improvement projects derived from analysis of patterns of care, and therefore required no special funding on the part of this contractor. Feedback to the author concerning the issues presented is welcomed.

A.D. Mims, M.D., MPH (✉)
Medicare Quality Improvement, Quality Improvement Organization, Alliant GMCF,
1455 Lincoln Parkway, Suite 800, Atlanta, GA 30331, USA

American Health Quality Association, 1725 I (Eye) Street, NW Suite 300,
Washington, DC 20006, USA
e-mail: Adrienne.mims@gmcf.org

J.C. Pederson, M.D., MS
Medical Affairs, Stratis Health, 2901 Metro Drive, Suite 400, Bloomington, MN 55425, USA
e-mail: jpederson@stratishealth.org

J.A. Gold, M.D., JD, MPH
MetaStar, Inc, 2909 Landmark Place, Madison, WI 53713, USA
e-mail: jgold@metastar.com

AHQA	American Health Quality Association
AHRQ	Agency for Healthcare Research and Quality
AMA-PCPI	American Medical Association – Physician Consortium for Performance Improvement
AMDA	American Medical Directors Association
BFCC	Beneficiary and Family Centered Care
CKD	Chronic Kidney Disease
CMO	Chief Medical Officer
CMS	Centers for Medicare and Medicaid Services
CORF	Comprehensive Outpatient Rehabilitation Facility
DOQ-IT	Doctor's Office Quality-Information Technology
EMCRO	Experimental Medical Care Review Organizations
EHR	Electronic Health Record
EMTALA	Emergency Medical Treatment and Labor Act
FY	Fiscal Year
HCFA	Health Care Financing Organization
HCQII	Health Care Quality Improvement Initiative
HCQIP	Health Care Quality Improvement Program
HHS	Health and Human Services
INTERACT	Interventions to Reduce Acute Care Transfers
IOM	Institute of Medicine
JAMA	Journal of the American Medical Association
LAN	Learning and Action Network
LANE	Local Area Networks for Excellence
NCQA-GMAP	National Committee Quality Assurance – Geriatric Measurement Advisory Panel
OPPS	Outpatient Prospective Payment System
PLN	Physician Leadership Network
PPACA	Patient Protection and Affordable Care Act
PQRS	Physician Quality Reporting System
PRO	Peer Review Organization
PSPC	Patient Safety and Clinical Pharmacy Services Collaborative
PSRO	Professional Standards Review Organization
QA	Quality Assurance
QAPI	Quality Assurance and Performance Improvement
QI	Quality Improvement
QIN	Quality Innovation Network
QIO	Quality Improvement Organization
RFP	Request for Proposals
SOW	Scope of Work or Statement of Work

Overview

The national Quality Improvement Organization (QIO) Program is administered by the Centers for Medicare and Medicaid Services (CMS), the Federal agency that administers Medicare, the federal portion of Medicaid, and other federal health insurance programs. QIOs are private, mostly not-for-profit organizations that hold contracts with CMS aimed at protecting the quality of health care available to Americans with Medicare. Historically, CMS contracted with one organization in each state as well as Washington D.C., Puerto Rico, and the U.S. Virgin Islands to serve as that state/jurisdiction's Quality Improvement Organization (QIO) contractor. QIO contracts have traditionally been 3 years in length, with each 3-year cycle referenced as an ordinal Scope or Statement of Work (SOW). (For instance, the contract cycle from 2011 to 2014 is known as the "10th SOW") [1]. Starting in 2014, CMS will engage contractors to serve as QIOs in 5-year cycles as parts of networks that span across the country, rather than stand-alone entities that work independently in a single state or territory [2]. This restructuring of the QIO Program will lead to many "flavors" of QIOs doing many different things, not limited to traditional quality improvement activities.

The statutory mission of the QIO Program is set forth in Title XI of the Social Security Act [3]. More specifically, Section 1154 of the Act states that the mission of the QIO Program is to improve the effectiveness, efficiency, economy, and quality of services delivered to Medicare beneficiaries and to ensure that those services are reasonable and necessary.

CMS identifies the core functions of the QIOs as:

- Improving quality of care for beneficiaries;
- Protecting the integrity of the Medicare Trust Fund by ensuring that Medicare pays only for services and goods that are reasonable and necessary and that are provided in the most appropriate setting; and
- Protecting beneficiaries by expeditiously addressing individual complaints, such as complaints from beneficiaries and their families about the quality of health care services they receive under Medicare, appeals from beneficiaries who believe an aspect of their care is ending prematurely (e.g., a premature hospital discharge), violations of the Emergency Medical Treatment and Labor Act (EMTALA), and related responsibilities as articulated in the law governing QIOs [1].

The QIO program impacts Medicare beneficiaries both on an individual basis and as a whole. In FY 2009 more than 45 million persons were covered by Medicare; that is 98.1 % of individuals aged 65 and older. Additionally, 7.3 million people with disabilities or end-stage renal disease were covered. These Medicare beneficiaries represent a significant portion of the nation's population (14.7 %), many of whom receive better, safer care in the thousands of hospitals, nursing homes, and other care settings where QIOs work [4].

Many current QIOs evolved from antecedent organizations with long histories of involvement in the Medicare peer review program. The next section offers an overview of the Medicare program's quality improvement efforts.

Background

Physicians have been essential to the development of the quality improvement initiatives since Medicare's inception. The Medicare statute first adopted in 1965 included language focused on patient safety and access to care from competent health care providers. In 1971, the U.S. Congress authorized Experimental Medical Care Review Organizations (EMCROs) to evaluate services provided to Medicare beneficiaries, with a focus on reducing unnecessary utilization of services through physician education and research. EMCROs, which operated from 1970 to 1974, were voluntary groups of physicians who received grants from the National Center for Health Services Research, a predecessor agency of the U.S. Agency for Healthcare Research and Quality (AHRQ) [5].

In 1972, an amendment was adopted to Title XI of the Social Security Act authorizing the establishment of Professional Standards Review Organizations (PSROs). The physician-sponsored PSROs used local physicians to evaluate cases to determine the medical necessity of services. The PSROs also focused on retrospective utilization review of hospital admissions and length of stay [5].

PSROs evolved to PROs thanks to the Peer Review Improvement Act of 1982. PROs, or Utilization and Quality Control Peer Review Organizations, launched in 1984 with a continued focus on retrospective case review along with educational or punitive measures for individual providers when needed. The Act continued to require significant physician participation, defining the PROs as physician-sponsored (10 % of local physicians participating as reviewers) or physician-access (at least one physician per specialty area to conduct medical reviews). Additional changes included not reviewing cases of close colleagues, having a consumer representative on the PRO Board of Directors, and the option of a for-profit status for the PRO. The statute provided for one PRO per state (50) and one each for Washington DC, Puerto Rico, and the Virgin Islands [5].

Funding for the PRO program originally came from annual appropriations. However, legislation starting in 1982 funded PRO work from the Medicare Trust Fund directly [5]. This stable funding source gave the Government the flexibility it needed to award contracts longer than 1 year. These longer contract periods evolved into cycles called Scopes of Work or SOWs, which distinguish each contract from the others. The 1st SOW went from 1984 to 1986 with a focus on reducing inappropriate hospital admissions. The 2nd SOW extended the PROs' mandatory quality monitoring and review activities to skilled nursing facilities, home health care agencies, hospital outpatient facilities, and physician office settings. The 2nd and 3rd SOWs continued to focus on retrospective case review that identified inappropriate care, but in isolated pockets on a case-by-case basis.

During the 3rd SOW contract cycle, PROs conducted random reviews of 25 % of all Medicare visits in their jurisdictions. A 1990 Institute of Medicine report [6] noted two glaring weaknesses of this approach: physician reviews were unreliable (i.e., studies in which cases were reviewed by other physicians frequently resulted in determinations different from the original ones), and PRO activity elicited substantial animosity from the medical community.

In response to these concerns, as well as to the growing evidence base for guidelines and processes that improve care, PROs began to shift their focus to building cooperative relationships with providers that attempted to improve care prospectively, rather than attempting to address quality issues once they happened.

In 1992, during the 3rd SOW, the Health Care Quality Improvement Initiative (HCQII) [7] redirected PROs to focus away from individual provider errors detected retrospectively towards evaluating practice patterns prospectively and using physician expertise to guide larger scale improvement at the institutional or national level [5]. HCQII would be followed by the Health Care Quality Improvement Program (HCQIP) in 1995, which positioned PROs as part of a comprehensive program that sought to unify and streamline quality improvement work across the Medicare and Medicaid programs (Table 2.1) [8].

The 4th and 5th SOWs (1993–1999) added quality improvement projects focused upon areas of high morbidity and mortality among Medicare beneficiaries where there existed strong scientific evidence that interventions could improve outcomes. Physicians were used as subject matter experts on strategies to impact the clinical topic areas of heart disease, diabetes, and preventive care. The government also called upon PROs to improve data collection and use of standardized measures to demonstrate statewide improvement. There was an emphasis on local collaboration among government, providers, and consumers to achieve desirable outcomes. Physicians became involved to build stakeholder relationships. During this period, PROs adopted practices from the growing literature surrounding quality improvement methodology, including introducing thousands of physician partners to the Plan-Do-Study-Act (PDSA) Cycle (the Shewhart Cycle), designed to implement changes in a clinical or administrative practice by making incrementally small-scale adjustments, and testing and learning from these adjustments before scaling the changes more widely. In addition to mandatory case review activities, there was a focus on beneficiary outreach and education [5].

Table 2.1 QIO contract cycles

Cycle	Date	Name	Responsible federal agency
1st SOW	1984–1986	Peer Review Organization (PRO) (starting in 1983)	Health Care Financing Administration (HCFA)
2nd SOW	1986–1989	PRO	HCFA
3rd SOW	1989–1993	PRO	HCFA
4th SOW	1993–1996	PRO	HCFA
5th SOW	1996–1999	PRO	HCFA
6th SOW	1999–2002	Name updated from PRO to Quality Improvement Organization (QIO) [9]	HCFA/Centers for Medicare and Medicaid Services (CMS)
7th SOW	2002–2005	QIO	CMS
8th SOW	2005–2008	QIO	CMS
9th SOW	2008–2011	QIO	CMS
10th SOW	2011–2014	QIO	CMS
11th SOW	2014–2019	QIO, though not necessarily state/territory based	CMS

In the 4th and 5th SOWs, individual PROs developed their own "local projects" to improve care. These projects were led by a physician Principal Clinical Coordinator and physician Associate Clinical Coordinators, who directed literature searches, measure development, choice of intervention, participant recruitment, analysis of results, and communication with participants. Starting with the 6th SOW, the topics and measures for most QIO quality improvement projects were determined centrally by CMS.

In 2002, CMS renamed PROs Quality Improvement Organizations or QIOs. The name change – aligned with the program's 20th anniversary – reflected Medicare's evolving emphasis on improving clinical quality of care, and the vital role that PROs (now QIOs) would play in making these improvements [9]. Clinical topics were added, including stroke and pneumonia with standardized indicators for the hospital, long-term care, and outpatient settings. Three local projects were required including one showing a reduction in disparity and one based on local needs. Physicians played a major role in designing these projects. The contract included a separate focus on working with Medicare+Choice (M+C) plans on two performance improvement projects. A portion of 6th SOW funding was set aside for special studies; more than 2,000 such projects were funded [5].

While national performance measurement of 6th SOW results noted national improvement in 20 out of 22 indicators for Medicare fee-for-service care [10], the 7th SOW (2002–2005) was designed to evaluate QIO performance based on achievement of specific state-level targets. Mandatory projects were included for home health agencies, nursing homes, managed care plans, and physician offices. Special attention was required for rural and underserved populations [11]. Participation by providers and practitioners in QI projects was voluntary. QIO physicians played a key role in the success of these projects, recruiting physician collaborators, enlisting professional associations to endorse the projects and inform their members of that endorsement, and offering medical support to internal teams [5].

At the turn of the millennium, CMS began to focus on making the rich data available in Medicare's files available to the public. CMS' efforts to increase transparency of quality information included launching the Nursing Home Compare website, a publicly available database on the Medicare.gov website aimed at sharing the results of quality measures with the general public and using these results to motivate beneficiaries to make smarter choices about their care options. Over the years, CMS also launched similar websites for home health agencies, hospitals, dialysis clinics, and physician practices. Increased involvement of Medicare beneficiaries occurred as they were added to panels advising the QIO project teams. QIOs provided hotlines and offered beneficiaries the option of having their complaints addressed through mediation rather than the longer formal case review process. CMS recognized a handful of QIOs as providing national-level expertise and leadership to support other QIOs for specific clinical topics or provider settings. These support centers served as peer-leaders among the QIO community as each specialized in one particular facet of QIO work, providing educational materials, compiling scientific evidence and tools, and convening educational sessions to distribute knowledge QIOs then could spread in their home states [5].

The 8th SOW (2005–2008) changed the focus from making incremental improvements on quality metrics as they apply to individual episodes of care to achieving transformational change in systems and processes (i.e., change that has broad, systemic impact). The Doctor's Office Quality-Information Technology (DOQ-IT) program was implemented nationally to promote the use of health information technology [5]. Many QIO physicians developed innovative projects to impact the quality of care through a new funding mechanism of special focus projects. One such project involved the development of Interventions to Reduce Acute Care Transfers (INTERACT), which focused on reducing the need for nursing home residents to receive acute-care hospital treatment. Over time, the lessons learned from the INTERACT program have led to innovations in how nursing homes coordinate care for their residents. One innovation in particular created new ways to share information among nursing home caregivers that encourages them to work more effectively together to identify, communicate, and evaluate changes in a resident's health or well-being – these early, proactive communication loops are vital to detecting potential problems early enough to avoid costly and disruptive hospital stays for residents [12].

After a series of QIO-specific recommendations from the IOM in 2006, CMS strengthened the QIO Program for the 9th SOW (2008–2011) by [4]:

- Strengthening evaluation design to better assess the impact of the Program;
- Strengthening financial oversight and establishing requirements for QIO board governance to assure appropriate use of contractor funds and the representation of key constituencies;
- Increasing competition for QIO contracts;
- Enabling QIOs to release information to beneficiaries about QIO findings related to their complaints;
- Focusing QIOs on achieving national quality goals aimed at improving care for beneficiaries with significant medical needs;
- Supporting local initiatives that develop and use information on quality and cost to help beneficiaries, their caregivers, and their health professionals make better choices about beneficiaries' care.

The 9th SOW (2008–2011) was administered through 53 contracts covering 50 states, Puerto Rico, the U.S. Virgin Islands, and Washington DC, awarded to 41 independent organizations that collectively employed about 2,300 individuals across the country. During Fiscal Year 2009, CMS spent $174.6 million to administer the program [4]. While they employed fewer physicians than in earlier years, every state had physicians in positions of leadership, case review, or consultation.

QIOs employed additional tools to monitor and report on their impact on the care provided in their states/jurisdictions. QIOs focused on providing intensive support to low-performing providers and practitioners. Roughly 85 % of the provider facilities that QIOs assisted were determined by CMS using CMS data. The QIOs chose the remaining 15 % [4].

The 9th SOW included as content areas for all QIOs: beneficiary protection including mandatory case review, patient safety in hospitals and nursing homes, primary prevention, early detection, and providing assistance in using EHRs. Three "Sub-National" projects were awarded competitively to a subset of QIOs: Chronic Kidney Disease (CKD); Care Transitions to Reduce Hospital Readmissions; and Reducing Health Disparities among Patients with Diabetes [4].

The 10th SOW (2011–2014) at this writing is being carried out by 37 contractors holding contracts for 50 states, Puerto Rico, the U.S. Virgin Islands, and Washington D.C., with a total contract value of approximately $200 million/year. The program has three aims: improving patient care, improving population health, and lowering health care costs through quality improvement. All three of these aims support the aims of the U.S. Department of Health and Human Services' National Quality Strategy. Through large-scale Learning and Action Networks, discussed below, QIOs accelerate the pace of change. Improvement initiatives encourage innovation and respond to community needs. The voice of the Medicare beneficiary is prominent in all activities. Initiatives are open to providers at all levels of clinical performance that make a commitment to improvement. Improvement initiatives include collaborative projects, online interaction, and peer-to-peer education. The QIOs support CMS's value-based purchasing programs with technical assistance to providers that includes sharing best practices, assisting with data analysis, and conducting improvement activities [13]. There are QIO physicians at all levels of local programs.

Focus areas include [13]:

- Protecting the rights of Medicare beneficiaries by reviewing complaints about the quality of care received and processing appeals of the denial or discontinuation of health care services.
- Facilitating patient safety initiatives in hospitals to reduce central line bloodstream infections, catheter-associated urinary tract infections, *Clostridium difficile* infections, and surgical site infections.
- Providing technical assistance for reporting inpatient and outpatient quality data to CMS.
- Working with nursing homes to reduce the prevalence of pressure ulcers, the use of physical restraints, and the use of antipsychotic medications for managing behavior in people with dementia; and providing technical assistance in implementing Quality Assurance and Performance Improvement or QAPI methodology to structure quality improvement projects in nursing homes.
- Decreasing the incidence of adverse drug events by bringing clinical pharmacists, physicians, and facilities together to participate in the national Patient Safety and Clinical Pharmacy Services Collaborative (PSPC).
- Reducing readmissions within 30 days of hospital discharge; changing processes of care at the community level in hospitals, home health agencies, dialysis facilities, nursing homes, and physician offices; and bringing together providers, patient advocacy organizations, and other stakeholders in community coalitions.
- Assisting physician practices in using their electronic health record systems to coordinate preventive services and report related quality measure data to CMS. Practices can participate in a Learning and Action Network focused on reducing patient risk factors for cardiac disease. QIOs partner with their local Health Information Technology Regional Extension Centers (RECs) to promote health IT integration into clinical practice.

The Patient Protection and Affordable Care Act (PPACA), called for the development of new models of care and the emergence of new models for reimbursement for medical claims payment [14]. New care delivery models include increased use of performance on quality measures to impact reimbursement (Accountable Care Organizations). The 10th SOW includes tasks to support providers to begin submitting PQRS data and to improve performance on those submitted measures.

Milestone changes to the structure of the QIO program in 2014 are a result of Section 261 of the Trade Adjustment Assistance Extension Act of 2011. The U.S. Secretary of Health and Human Services was given the authority to contract with a broader array of entities than in the past, which may result in multistate entities providing local QI support, rather than a state-by-state approach to QIO work [15]. As a result, broad changes will occur in subsequent contracts [2].

- The contract cycle moves from 3 years to 5 years.
- Fewer organizations will coordinate activities over several states.
- CMS will award medical case review for Medicare beneficiaries to Beneficiary- and Family-Centered Care Quality Improvement Organizations (BFCC-QIOs), while quality improvement work will be conducted by Quality Innovation Network QIOs (QIN-QIOs). Thus, the traditional work of the QIO Program will be performed by different types of QIOs across the country, rather than assigning all QIO work to a single organization within a single state.

Physician leadership will be invaluable to improving quality of care on a multi-state level, while local physician involvement for recruitment, convening advisory boards, stakeholder interactions, clinical education sessions, and design of implementation tools and strategies will be essential for successful quality improvement at the community level.

Capabilities of QIOs

As noted, the QIOs' charge from CMS has become increasing complex, as CMS tasks QIOs with supporting more provider venues and changing the program's strategies, and at the same time introducing technology to effect change. In order to provide services as a QIO, an organization needs the capability to implement quality improvement initiatives at a statewide and a local community level, as well as across states. QIO staff expertise includes (Table 2.2):

Table 2.2 Capabilities of staff working at the QIO

Technical assistance	Public speaking	Process redesign
QI methodologies	Community organizing	Government contracting
Data analysis and reporting	Technical writing	Clinical practice
Information technology	Change management	Recruitment
Electronic health record systems	Communications and publication	Convening and managing a collaborative
Evaluation	Security	Outreach
Clinician and patient education	Contract management	Data collection

Thus the QIO physician will work with an interdisciplinary team of individuals with a range of expertise that differs from a clinical practice or educational environment.

The Work of QIOs

The QIO Program's primary purpose is to improve the quality of care provided to Medicare beneficiaries. It does this in a two-fold way. First, the QIO provides a mechanism for Medicare beneficiaries and their representatives to raise concerns regarding the quality of the care they have received. Second, the QIO supports providers in improving the quality of care they deliver to their patients. Physicians have a comprehensive view on how various aspects of the healthcare system impact the patient and thus can play an essential role in improvement efforts within the QIO.

An understanding of the general difference between quality assurance (QA) and quality improvement (QI) provides the basis for a good understanding of the purview of the QIO Program. QA typically focuses on variation in practice – especially variation in practice that would result in falling below the generally accepted standard of care or the minimal standard of care. QI typically focuses on setting goals and striving to improve performance. Goals are chosen based on the perceived gap between current performance and what it felt to be "best practice" derived from what is known from medical literature or what is observed and measured in the practice setting. QI generally assumes a goal of meeting the standard of care and therefore goals are selected based on a desire to meet or exceed the current performance or benchmarks set by the high performers. QI is therefore a continuous process as the standard of care and best practice is always evolving and improving. These concepts of QA and QI are evident in both major bodies of QIO work: beneficiary and family centered care (BFCC) and quality improvement (QI).

Also important to an understanding of the work of the QIO are the concepts of "systems" and "processes." A basic definition of a process is the series of steps that are taken in order to complete a task or an action. The term "system" refers a combination of multiple processes. Health care is made up of many systems and these systems are in turn made up of many processes. For example, in settings of care where medications are administered, such as hospitals or long-term care facilities, there exists a system for medication administration that includes all the processes involved in taking a medication from the point of prescribing to administering it to a patient. Both QA and QI focus on systems and processes in order to assess causes of variation and to look for breakdowns or determine opportunities for improvement. An example of this in the QIO program is the work that has been done to decrease the prevalence and incidence of pressure ulcers in the hospital and long-term care settings. The focus in eliminating pressure ulcers has been on the system of care and the processes aimed at assuring appropriate preventive measures are taken to preserve skin integrity for each patient at the right time.

A basic assumption of both QA and QI is that the outcomes that are achieved in health care are influenced most by the systems and processes that lead to those outcomes, and it is these systems and processes that influence the individual behavior of those who engage in those processes. Any given process permits certain results and precludes certain other results. Thus, individual behavior can achieve certain outcomes only if the process permits these outcomes. The systems and processes that individuals work within are usually a much stronger determining factor in outcomes than individual activity. Therefore, in both QA and QI, if we are working to change an outcome, in the vast majority of cases this needs to be done through changing the systems and processes. This philosophy is evident in the work of the QIO. It is often assumed that improvement in quality is achieved through education. While education is important and part of all QA and QI work, it is often not sufficient. The QIO plays a unique role in helping providers understand that frequently individuals providing care have all needed knowledge and skill; however, it is the systems and processes that prevent those individuals from delivering the right care at all times for all patients. This approach requires taking time up front to understand the systems and processes; however, ultimately this step can save time by reducing rework, and in the end will produce a better outcome that is more likely to be sustained over time. This approach is also one of the reasons QIO work is rewarding to QIO physicians.

The QIO approaches improving quality of systems and processes from two vantage points; case-based that uses information gained from individual episodes of care, and setting-based that looks at care provide in a setting or across settings. The case-based approach is most evident in the BFCC-focused work that addresses variation in quality, coding and utilization through review of the medical records that document individual patients' episodes of care. The setting-based approach is evident in the QI initiatives that focus on the various settings of care such as hospital, outpatient, and long-term care. In this approach the QIO is not focused in individual episodes of care but instead in looking at aggregate data such as publicly reported measures of care.

The BFCC-QIO uses information found through review of episodes of care with the input of patients, patient representatives, and providers to identify opportunities to improve the quality of care provided and address utilization issues. Because most of the episodes of care QIOs review come to them from complaints or appeals from Medicare beneficiaries or their families, BFCC work gives voice to those receiving care. In its review, the QIO aims to ensure that this voice is heard to improve care, not just for that beneficiary, but for all patients in similar care situations. As they do this, QIOs review the quality of care in the context of practice guidelines, the current evidence base, and the community standard of practice.

Physicians play a central role in the BFCC work. Often the review of an episode of care will begin with Medicare beneficiaries raising a concern over care they have received or requesting a review when their benefits have been terminated, which occurs upon discharge from the hospital or other setting of care that is paid by Medicare Part A. The QIO staff work with the beneficiaries to understand their concerns and determine if they can be addressed by the QIO. The key source of data the QIO uses for the BFCC work is medical record documentation. Although the actual review of the medical record is done by outside physicians that are matched to the case by specialty and geography, the QIO physician makes certain the reviews are consistent not only with evidence but across reviews. This typically requires spending time reviewing each case and discussing the case with the physician reviewer as well as the Medicare beneficiary or family and the provider(s) involved in the care.

The range of case types included in the BFCC QIO work includes:

- Appeals for termination of benefits in any setting that is paid by Medicare; acute inpatient, long-term care hospitals, skilled nursing facilities, Comprehensive Outpatient Rehabilitation Facilities (CORFs), and hospice. In these reviews the QIO is asked to determine if it is appropriate for Part A Medicare coverage to end. This involves reviewing the medical record to determine if the beneficiary was ready for discharge or if s/he still required the services that could only be provided in that setting.
- Requests for higher weighted DRG's. These reviews are requested by a hospital after a patient has been discharged to determine from a clinical standpoint whether the hospital is eligible for a higher reimbursement.
- EMTALA (Emergency Medical Treatment and Labor Act) referrals. The QIO reviews the medical information for CMS to make the clinical determination as to whether a violation of EMTALA exists.
- Quality of Care concerns. These reviews arise when Medicare beneficiaries or their representatives contact the QIO because they feel the care they received was not appropriate or was harmful. They also arise out of utilization reviews as each record reviewed by the QIO is also evaluated for quality of care concerns.

The BFCC work can be personally and professionally rewarding for the QIO staff physician and for the physicians who perform the medical record reviews. In the process of performing the review and analyzing the results, physicians improve their own knowledge and skills, directly impact the care Medicare beneficiaries receive, and work directly with providers to help them determine ways to change their systems and processes of care in order to provide the high quality care they desire for their patients.

The QI QIO work has evolved over the years and continues to evolve. As noted in the background section, the clinical topics that the QIOs are asked to address change based on CMS's analysis of national performance data. Each QIO is asked to work on these topics and to elicit improvements. CMS lays out the general approach and the contract deliverables; however, the approach to achieving improvement is determined by the QIO taking into account the local health care systems and environment.

One way QIOs have worked to identify high performing organizations and to rapidly share effective practices is through learning and action networks (LANs). These LANs are topic-focused and can be statewide, across multiple states, or within a specific community. The idea behind LANs is that they connect organizations and individuals that have similar goals for QI in a collaborative effort where everyone teaches and everyone learns. The intended result of these LANs is rapid, wide-scale improvement that would not happen with each organization working independently. An example of this work is highlighted in an article published in the Journal of the American Medical Association (JAMA) that showed that hospitalizations and re-hospitalizations among Medicare patients declined nearly twice as much in communities where Quality Improvement Organizations (QIOs) coordinated interventions that engaged whole communities to improve care than in comparison communities [16]. This result was achieved through:

- Developing effective community coalitions involving hospitals, nursing facilities, home care, hospice agencies, physicians and local agencies to meet clinical and social service needs that may prevent patients from getting or staying well;
- Generating and implementing standard transition processes across all local health care settings;
- Transferring patient clinical information among providers in a timely and effective way;
- Helping patients and their family members become actively engaged in their transitions by keeping a personal record, knowing the 'red flags' for trouble, ensuring they receive the right medications, and follow-through on appropriate follow-up care.

Besides highlighting the cross-setting work of the QIO, this coordinated effort also highlights the important role of the physician in QIO work. In each of the above approaches the physician plays a critical role in developing strategy and education, and facilitating communication among various providers.

In addition to the LANs, the QI work also involves direct technical assistance to providers, which involves consultation and hands-on teaching. This approach has been evident in the work QIOs have done in the long-term care setting aimed at clinical topics such as the reduction of physical restraints, and other topics such as the provisions of the Affordable Care Act that require each nursing home to implement its own Quality Assurance and Performance Improvement (QAPI) plan. In these cases, QIO staff and physicians will work one-on-one with facilities to teach QI skills, review data, help with implementation of improvement interventions, and measure effectiveness. Physicians practicing in the community or within the organizations working with the QIO can be an effective resource to support the work of the QIO and provide ongoing education and support to quality improvement initiatives. The QIOs strive to engage physicians and value their support.

Depending on the needs of the state, QIO work may also focus on specific populations such as rural providers or underserved communities, with multicultural activities aimed at meeting the needs of a changing Medicare demographic.

Role of the Physician in the QIO

QIOs have typically employed physicians to serve either as medical director for the BFCC work or as a clinical and quality improvement leader for the QI work. Taking a position in a QIO can be very rewarding but is also very different from clinical practice. One of the biggest rewards QIO physicians receive is being able

Table 2.3 Roles of physicians working in a QIO

Medical Reviewer	Medical Director	Subject Matter Expert Consultant
Chief Medical Officer	Chief Executive Officer	Senior Vice President
Associate Medical Director	Director of Research	Principal Clinical Coordinator
Director of Medical Affairs	State Program Director	Chief Medical Information Officer

to impact the health and well-being of people on a larger scale than is possible in the individual clinical setting. In a clinical practice, physicians have the opportunity to work with each patient individually to work toward maintaining or improving their health or quality of life. See Table 2.3 of examples of roles for physicians in the QIO program.

Skills Needed

Although clinical training, knowledge and experience are essential for a physician to be successful in QIO work, these skills are not sufficient for success. In many QIOs, the physician is an integral part of the leadership team and also has a hand-on role in BFCC or the various QI initiatives. From a recent survey of physicians working at QIOs, it was noted that 80 % completing the survey have an additional relevant degree or certifications including MPH, MS, MSPH, JD, PhD, MHA, MMA, and MBA. Some of the additional skills needed to be successful in the QIO physician role include:

- Systems and critical thinking: This is the most important skill because of the QIO focus on systems and processes. The QIO physician must be able to model and teach such thinking. An example would be leading a root cause analysis (RCA) with the goal of not only helping the provider identify the root cause of a problem, but also teaching the provider how to use the RCA process for future work.
- QI tools and techniques: There are a number of tools and techniques that assist in quality improvement work and support systems thinking. The QIO physician must be able to model and teach these tools and techniques. An example of this is helping providers understand the use of the Plan-Do- Study-Act (PDSA or Shewhart) cycle and the power of small tests of change. Helping providers use this technique can allow them to make rapid improvements.
- Analytic skills: Although QIOs typically employ various other kinds of professionals to assist, it is important that physicians be able to understand, interpret and transfer the results to be clinically relevant
- Teamwork: Much of the work at a QIO is done in teams. Therefore, the QIO physician needs to be able both to lead and to participate in teams. In addition, the QIO physician will be called upon to teach team skills to other providers as part of basic quality improvement skills.
- Creativity: Although CMS provides the general approach for the QI work, the specific approach is left to the states. QIO physicians need to use their knowledge

of the local health care environment and current state initiatives to find new and innovative ways to address gaps and to encourage improvement.
- Communication: QIO physicians have numerous opportunities to speak in front of a variety of audiences, so good presentation skills are essential. It is also important to have good writing skills and be able to translate information into language that resonates with a wide range of readers, from other physicians to Medicare beneficiaries and their families.
- Networking: A big part of the QIO physician job is building relationships with physicians and others to understand current needs and trends and to gain support for quality initiatives. This may involve participating on local organizations, committees or work groups as well as being active in national stakeholder and partner events.
- Education: QIO physicians are often asked to lead educational sessions on a variety of topics. This requires the ability effectively to utilize adult education principles in order to maximize the impact of education on actual systems, processes, and outcomes of care. An example is teaching a group of physicians how to lead RCA teams. This requires leading them through hands-on activities to gain experience with the tools and techniques that constitute the RCA process.

In summary, given the scope of the QIO work and the skills required, becoming a physician in a QIO can be personally and professionally rewarding as well as intellectually challenging. Success requires gaining skills and competencies beyond those of a successful clinician. There are few opportunities where physicians can affect the health care provided in their state to the degree they can by working for the QIO. Such a position allows physicians to gain knowledge and understanding of the health care industry, and to interact with regulators and policymakers at a state and national level as well as with other partners and stakeholders. Furthermore, a successful QIO experience can be an excellent training for other positions.

Stakeholder Engagement

Quality improvement work is complex and multifactorial. In order to be successful, a project needs both support and input from a variety of viewpoints. To that end, it is essential to develop and maintain ongoing relationships with stakeholders, so that when collaborative engagement is needed, support is easier to garner. Potential stakeholder organizations include the state associations for physicians, nurses, pharmacists, hospitals, nursing homes, hospice, assisted living, state survey agency, AARP, Alzheimer's disease, state public and private agencies including Area Agencies on Aging, CMS, Medicaid, public health, Health Information Technology Regional Extension Centers (RECs), private insurance carriers, and schools of medicine, public health, health policy, pharmacy, and gerontology.

Whether the project is facility-based, local, statewide, or multi-state in scope, the QIO physician can be integral in negotiating collaborative relationships. With a background of interdisciplinary team work for care plan development, comprehensive assessment, and case management, with patients eligible for Medicare, geriatricians are uniquely suitable for working in this environment. Engaging and valuing the unique contribution of team members as equal contributors is an important skill in team leaders and members.

Within a facility, a quality improvement team typically consists of individuals from different backgrounds who are affected by a process. For example, in the hospital setting, working on a project to improve infection control, the team may include a hospitalist, surgeon, nurse, operating room technician, pharmacist, or specialist in utilization review, infection control, risk management, laboratory, discharge planning, environmental services, or patient education. In a long term care environment, a project to reduce pressure ulcers could include, a medical director, director of nursing, admission nurse, nursing assistant, dietician, wound care nurse, physical therapist, pharmacist, environmental services specialist, social worker, and ombudsman.

Quality improvement projects affecting a broader community may include the oversight of an advisory board. One example is an effort in Georgia to reduce statewide rates of inappropriate antipsychotic medication in patients with dementia in long term care facilities. For this quality improvement project, a multi-organizational effort was needed. In Georgia, the baseline rates for antipsychotic use in dementia for long stay residents was one of the highest in the nation in 2011 [17]. The state set a goal of a 15 % reduction in use by 12/31/12, identical to the national goal [17]. The Advancing Excellence in America's Nursing Homes Campaign supports statewide coalitions of stakeholders called Local Area Networks for Excellence (LANEs) [18]. The Georgia QIO co-convened an advisory board to guide this effort along with the state LANE under the leadership of a QIO geriatrician. The advisory board consisted of representatives from the regional CMS office, the state nursing home association, geriatric pharmacy, geriatric psychiatry, geriatric medicine, state survey agency, geriatric nurse practitioner, long term care pharmacy, occupational therapy, activity director, Alzheimer's Association, ombudsman, and quality improvement specialist. As a result of an intensive, focused effort, the statewide rates dropped surpassing the goal of 15 %, resulting in a 20 % reduction [19].

On a national level, QIO physicians provide quality improvement expertise in a variety of organizations, workgroups, and technical expert panels. A survey of physicians working in the QIO program in 2013 found that they held positions with many organizations that impact the breadth of medical care across the country (Table 2.4).

Table 2.4 Affiliations of QIO physicians

American Geriatric Society (AGS)	American College of Physicians (ACP)	American Academy of Family Physicians (AAFP)
Medical school or residency programs; faculty appointments	National Committee for Quality Assurance – Geriatric Measurement Advisory Panel (NCQA-GMAP)	American Medical Association- Physician Consortium for Performance Improvement (AMA-PCPI)
American Cancer Society	State and County Medical Associations	Technical Expert Panels for CMS and others
Health Insurance Plan	American Medical Director Association	National Quality Forum

Trade Association

The national Quality Improvement Organization program is supported on a national level through a membership organization, the American Health Quality Association (AHQA) [20]. AHQA serves as a voice to represent organizations holding QIO contracts as they interact with HHS, CMS, Congress, and national associations. QIO physicians have held leadership positions within AHQA including President, members of the Board of Directors, chair of Advisory Committees, Networks, and expert panels.

Through AHQA, QIO physicians have served as a resource for Congressional leaders, government regulators, national organizations, and collaborators within the QIO program. Over the years, QIO physicians have met frequently with members of Congress, educating them about the quality improvement work of projects in their district and the needs of clinicians, patients, and facilities in their states. AHQA coordinates QIO physician input into the feedback solicitation process for the QIO contract, proposed rules, National Quality Forum proposed measures, and other national organizations' calls for input.

In the fall of 2012 into early 2013, a special focus committee including QIO physicians collaborated with HHS to help develop recommendations for measurement for the National Quality Strategy 2013 and influenced the CMS Quality Strategy 2013. In the fall of 2013, QIO physicians, pharmacist and quality improvement specialists provided input to the HHS National Action Plan for Adverse Drug Event Prevention [21] regarding measures to improve the safe use of medications for diabetes, anticoagulation, and pain management.

AHQA hosts a collaborative effort of QIO physicians called the Physician Leadership Network (PLN), which consists of physicians holding a variety of positions in their QIOs. Monthly conference calls and periodic onsite meetings have served as vehicles for information exchange, troubleshooting, program concerns, and the sharing of best practices. One product of the PLN was the development of a Clinical Discussion Series of webinars showcasing best practices on clinical topics important in the world of quality improvement [22]. The series demonstrates the interdisciplinary nature of the teamwork used in the QIO program in its production, presentation and attendance, and the importance of physician leadership.

Conclusion

Physicians choosing to build a career or work as consultants within the QIO arena can find that they are able to use a variety of skills in addition to those of the clinical, teaching or research setting. Leadership and collaborative roles among QIO interdisciplinary teams for quality improvement or executive management can be very rewarding as a career path. Physicians interested in working with QIOs should contact the one covering their state and discuss areas of interest including medical review, participation in quality improvement activities, providing educational lectures, or collaborating on submitting a grant proposal.

Acknowledgment The authors are grateful to Centers for Medicare and Medicaid Services staff who reviewed the manuscript.

References

1. CMS website. http://www.cms.gov/Medicare/Quality-Initiatives-Patient-Assessment-Instruments/QualityImprovementOrgs/Future.html
2. FedBIZ QIN-QIO RFP. Available from: https://www.fbo.gov/index?s=opportunity&mode=form&id=dff522bababb6b9859bb783c08db6074
3. Title XI Social Security Act, section 1154. Available from: http://www.ssa.gov/OP_Home/ssact/title11/1154.htm
4. Report to Congress on the administration, cost, and impact of the Quality Improvement Organization (QIO) program for medicare beneficiaries for Fiscal Year (FY); 2009.
5. Medicare's Quality Improvement Organization program: maximizing potential. Pathways to quality health care. Available from: http://www.nap.edu/catalog/11604.html
6. Institute of Medicine. Medicare: a strategy for quality assurance, volume I. Washington, DC: The National Academies Press, 1990.
7. Jencks SF, Wilensky GR. The health care quality improvement initiative: a new approach to quality assurance in Medicare. JAMA. 1992;268(7):900–3.
8. Gagel BJ. Health care quality improvement program: a new approach. Healthcare Financ Rev. 1995;16(4):15–23.
9. 67 FR 36539 (24 May 2002).
10. Jencks SF, Huff ED, Cuerdon T. Change in the quality of care delivered to Medicare beneficiaries, 1998–1999 to 2000–2001. JAMA. 2003;289(3):305–12.
11. Rollow W, Lied TR, McGann P, Poyer J, LaVoie L, Kambic T, Bratzler DW, Ma A, Huff ED, Ramunno LD. Assessment of the Medicare Quality Improvement Organization program. Ann Intern Med. 2006;145(5):342–53.
12. http://interact2.net/index.aspx
13. QIO 10th SOW fact sheet. Available from: http://www.cms.gov/Medicare/Quality-Initiatives-Patient-Assessment-Instruments/QualityImprovementOrgs/Downloads/QIOOverview.pdf
14. The Patient Protection and Affordable Care Act. Available from: http://www.gpo.gov/fdsys/pkg/BILLS-111hr3590enr/pdf/BILLS-111hr3590enr.pdf
15. H.R.2832: Trade Adjustment Assistance Extension Act of 2011 – U.S. Available from: http://www.gpo.gov/fdsys/pkg/BILLS-112hr2832enr/pdf/BILLS-112hr2832enr.pdf
16. Brock J, Mitchell J, Irby K, Stevens B, Archibald T, Goroski A, Lynn J. Association between quality improvement for care transitions in communities and rehospitalizations among Medicare beneficiaries. JAMA. 2013;309(4):381.
17. Advancing Excellence quality website. Available from: http://www.nhqualitycampaign.org/files/Reducing_Inappropriate_Use_of_Antipsychotics_in_Nursing_Homes_part_2.pdf.slide 25 of 55
18. Advancing Excellence LANE. Available from: http://www.nhqualitycampaign.org/star_index.aspx?controls=lanes
19. CMS News. New data show antipsychotic drug use is down in nursing homes nationwide. Available from: http://www.nhqualitycampaign.org/files/dementia_care_release_FINAL.PDF

20. www.ahqa.org
21. HHS National Action Plan for Adverse Drug Event Prevention. Available from: https://www.federalregister.gov/articles/2013/09/04/2013-21434/solicitation-of-written-comments-on-draft-national-action-plan-for-adverse-drug-event-prevention
22. AHQA PLN webinar series website. Available from: http://www.ahqa.org/quality-improvement-organizations/physician-leadership-network

Chapter 3
Leadership Opportunities for Physicians

Laurie G. Jacobs

> *A leader takes people where they want to go. A great leader takes people where they don't necessarily want to go, but ought to be.*
>
> – Rosalynn Carter

Introduction

The Affordable Care Act and other economic and social forces are transforming the United States (US) health care system, and particularly the practice of medicine. Patients and physicians alike are apprehensive about the rapid rate and structure of these changes despite widespread ongoing public discussion of access, quality and cost in health care. Physicians who can lead and manage system change are increasingly in demand. They provide a vision for the future, design processes and systems of care, supervise the provision of care, assess the goals and quality of such care, manage physician performance, and direct investments in technology used in health care. They lead the way, bringing health care providers and patients along with them. Although leadership training and management skills are not standard components of a medical education, expertise in these areas can be developed through both informal and formal activities, training and education. This chapter will describe (1) definitions of leadership, (2) leadership styles, and, (3) operationalizing physician leadership to be responsive to local needs.

L.G. Jacobs, M.D. (✉)
Department of Medicine, Montefiore Medical Center and Albert Einstein College of Medicine, 111 East 210 Street, Bronx, NY 10467, USA
e-mail: lajacobs@montefiore.org

Defining Leadership

The definition of leadership is nuanced and complex. It is often easier to say what it is not – leadership is not simply characterized by the ability to manage people (John P. Kotter), a certain personality, a title, or an appointment. Effective leaders provide inspiration; they influence others (John Maxwell), set a direction (Peter Drucker), empower others (Bill Gates) and engage others to follow their vision (Warren Bennis). "Leadership is a process of social influence, which maximizes the efforts of others, towards the achievement of a goal," opines Kevin Kruse of Forbes Magazine [1]. Leaders deal with change, shape the future, motivate and inspire. Kruse emphasizes social influence, rather than power or title, which focuses on a goal, not influence for its own sake. Physician leaders are, at their essence, no different from other leaders.

Physician leaders embody the culture of a healthcare organization. They establish, emulate and communicate the organization's mission, core values and the motivation behind its programs. They help physicians, executives, staff, the board of trustees, and the public understand its values and how those values drive goals, strategies and programs. Physician leaders provide vision, motivation, training, and encouragement to their physicians and staff, and create an atmosphere in which they are heard, feel valued, and can succeed.

Equally, the physician leader must communicate the core values to external stakeholders: to patients and their families, to the community, and often, to a wider public arena, as healthcare organizations merge and grow. These other parties must also feel valued and believe that they have a voice in the direction of the organization that serves their community.

For example, one urban safety-net hospital may value improvement in primary care measures and the health status of its community and develop programs accordingly. An academic medical center may value advancing scientific knowledge and pursue growth of its basic and clinical research programs. Another organization may value clinical innovation and pursue the provision of specialized tertiary care for a specific disease, such as cancer, or for a special population, such as a children's hospital. None of these are mutually exclusive, but resources are usually limited and not all values and goals can be pursued. Choices must be made. A physician leader should participate in identifying institutional core values, selecting immediate and long-term goals, and designing the strategic plan to pursue those values and goals. Among other roles, the physician leader must provide affiliated physicians with clear performance objectives and expectations for the quality and conduct of care in pursuit of those values and goals. If the core values of an institution do not resonate with a physician leader, it may present a poor match for a leadership position.

Physicians are a challenging group of individuals to lead. They are highly educated and skilled professionals who are trained to think analytically. Physicians tend to value independence and autonomy, while their leaders must stimulate their fidelity to the mission, vision, core values and strategic direction of the healthcare organization. Leaders must be able to listen and promote discussion, and ultimately make timely decisions based upon their own analyses of the issues, while engendering the support of those being led.

Although leadership is not simply management, physician leaders may also assume management roles. Leadership is providing the vision for the future, and bringing others to work towards that vision. Management is identifying the way in which those being led will get there and overseeing that journey. Managers plan, organize, prepare budgets, evaluate, control and solve problems. Planning may be at any level from assessing the needs of a practice for additional space or clinical services, for example, to planning acquisitions of medical groups, new health policy and reimbursement schemes. Physician managers are often responsible for peer review, clinical productivity, quality, scope and conduct of clinical activity. They solve problems encountered by patients, providers, staff and others.

In evaluating physician leaders, one must assess their ability to lead separately from their skills as managers. Some physician leaders may possess equal strengths and ability in both areas, but that is rare. A leader must be able to identify and empower individuals who have management skills to complement his or her leadership in order to ultimately succeed.

Leaders are often described as agents of change. Although change is threatening, it is inevitable, proceeding with ever-increasing speed as technological innovation provides access to information and data, drives social integration, and alters the financial and political landscape. The healthcare arena is no different, and physician leaders are often chosen to be agents of change because of their professional stature and clinical expertise. Change may be in the form of new reimbursement methodologies and the need to assess various quality metrics when a medical group participates in an ACO, or at a system level. Leaders also create and initiate new modes of care, program evaluations, and methods to improve care through training, systems and programs.

Characteristics of Good Leaders

Emotional Intelligence

Physician leaders must engender respect from other physicians, patients and administrators, as well as demonstrate intellect, knowledge, familiarity with and skill in providing clinical care. Most successful leaders must also possess "emotional intelligence," a term coined by Daniel Goleman [2], which describes self-management skills and the ability to relate to others through empathy and social skills. Emotional intelligence, he asserts, plays an increasingly important role in successful leadership at higher levels of an organization where differences in technical skills are of lesser importance. Although technical skill is more highly valued in medicine, as physician leaders acknowledge, emotional intelligence is a more critical skill for the leader than specific technical expertise.

Goleman defines self-management as self-awareness, self-regulation (the ability to control impulses in behavior) and motivation, the passion for achievement. Many leaders fail because they lack one or another of these traits. Leaders who have a high degree of self-awareness know their strengths and failings and have a sense of when and how their emotions influence their responses and decisions. They can balance their capacity to be positive and encouraging as well as critical. One example of self-awareness is a physician leader who knows he performs poorly under time pressure and therefore controls his schedule to accommodate for preparation time. Another example of self-awareness and self-regulation in the management of other physicians is the common situation in which another physician in group meetings routinely speaks out in opposition to the leader's position, often using an extreme example as the norm for any problem. This behavior may antagonize and threaten leaders, causing them to respond defensively without thinking first. A leader with high emotional intelligence can allow the physician to speak, avoid becoming defensive, and also prevent the physician from derailing the discussion from the intended agenda. He/she may acknowledge the comment, and indicate that the group can return to it, time permitting. Common behaviors demonstrating poor self-awareness and regulation include constantly looking at or texting on cell phones during meetings, negative patient encounters, or routine lateness to clinical sessions.

Empathy and social skills are also critical to success as a physician leader. Empathy for those being led may be, in some ways, analogous to empathy that physicians demonstrate with patients. Leaders must be able to listen, most importantly, and be responsive to feedback and suggestions. In addition, a leader is often privy to the private lives and stresses of those being led. The leader must demonstrate that s/he cares while retaining a professional distance and confidentiality. Empathy and social skills are critical to problem solving, evaluation and feedback, interviewing, recruitment, and negotiation. The leader's skills must include ability to listen, be flexible, find appropriate resources and incentives at any juncture. Strength in this area engenders personal respect for leaders beyond what may pertain to their position and responsibilities. These components of emotional intelligence enable leaders to listen, make decisions, and persuade others to follow them in a new direction. Strong emotional intelligence also enables physician leaders to address behavioral and performance issues in others with both empathy and professionalism.

Personality Types

The personality characteristics of leaders in the military, political and business arena have been described throughout history and in the literature. The Myers-Briggs Type Indicator [3] is a tool that has been used for several decades to assess personality types based preferences. Physicians' preferences in selection of their clinical specialty has been characterized using this tool [4, 5]. The Myers-Briggs Type Indicator characterizes an individual's personality into 16 different types based upon four sets of opposite preferences: how individuals focus their attention and energy (extraversion [E] versus introversion [I]), how individuals prefer to take in information (sensing [S] versus iNtuition [N]), how people make decisions (thinking [T] versus feeling [F]), and finally, how people deal with the world (judging [J] versus perceiving [P]).

Eighty-five percent of executives have been found to have a combined preference for thinking and judging (TJ); the majority are characterized as introversion/sensing/thinking/judging (ISTJ 32 %) or extroversion/sensing/thinking/judging (ESTJ 28 %) personality types [6]. Physicians' responses on the Myers-Briggs Type Indicator most often categorize them as thinking/judging, in contrast to the general population in whom only half fall into this grouping. Differences between the personality style of physicians and that of their patients has been examined with regard to the effectiveness of doctor-patient communication. There is no data on physician leaders as a group. One might postulate that if there was significant congruence in personality preferences between physicians and their leaders, their communication and leadership may be more successful, but this has not been studied.

The Myers-Briggs Type Indicator can provide insight into one's personality preferences. It can also highlight areas in which one may lack awareness, called "blind spots." The Myers-Briggs Type Indicator is available online and is a useful exercise for physician leaders to assist in recognizing their personality style and their strengths and weaknesses.

How to Lead

The need to inspire, provide vision, garner trust and respect, as well as manage change, however, is not unique to physician leadership. James Gorman, Chairman and Chief Executive Officer of Morgan Stanley and Company, offered to new executives this list of "eight pieces of leadership advice" [7] which is equally relevant to physician leaders:

1. People follow simplicity. Offer guidance that tells your team what really matters and what you are shooting for.
2. Take calculated risks.
3. Have a plan. During crisis moments, people listen to the calm leader.
4. Stay fit, mentally and physically.
5. Be willing to make decisions with imperfect information and under time constraints. Then move forward to the next decision.
6. Bring together team members whose blended strengths make up for your weaknesses.
7. Find a work-life balance that suits you.
8. Don't follow the career path based on what your friends think.

One might add a few more items to the list:

9. Don't reveal all, but when doing so, always tell the truth; it is easier to remember
10. When explaining, try to use the same words, confusion may ensue from saying the same thing in different words
11. Try to occupy "the high ground," then recruit others to it
12. Encourage discussion, listen, and then make decisions promptly based upon your judgment

Leadership Styles

Goleman [8] also described several leadership styles which are familiar to all from historical figures: coercive, authoritative, affiliative, democratic, pacesetting and coaching. Although one would think that there is a preference in healthcare organizations which rely on teamwork to have leaders who embody the affiliative, democratic, or pacesetting style, this is far from universal. Often a leadership role is filled by convenience, politically motivated, or someone is chosen due to a dominant personality style which either compliments or is comfortable for other leaders in the organization. Thus it is important to understand various leadership styles when recruiting leaders as well as physician leaders working with organizational administrative leaders.

Those who are coercive expect behavior to strictly follow directions – "do what I tell you" – sometimes with an implied threat for lack of adherence. Political dictators or fascists come to mind. The responsibility to identify a plan and generate new ideas rests solely with the leader; flexibility and shared responsibility are not allowed. This style may be the most effective in a crisis situation such as running a code, or dealing with an epidemic or a disaster, when rapid decisions must be made and immediate compliance is required.

An authoritative leader presents a vision which is so compelling that individuals will follow. The vision must have clarity and indicate the individual's role in the larger group without the sense that they are commanded to follow under a coercive leader. Positive and negative examples might include strong religious leaders or leader of a cult religion. This leadership style can be as effective or destructive as the coercive style.

Leaders who employ the affiliative style attempt to build bridges to those being led, provide harmony and emotional ties, and create an atmosphere of "kumbaya".[1] This style may be most effective during times of stress or following a loss. It builds communication and loyalty but may not provide sufficient direction to team

---

[1] Kumbaya is a spiritual song from the 1930s. It became a standard campfire song in Scouting and summer camps, and enjoyed broader popularity during the folk revival of the 1960s. The song was originally associated with human and spiritual unity, closeness and compassion.... Available at: http://en.wikipedia.org/wiki/Kumbaya. Accessed 21 Aug 2013.

members when employed as a sole leadership style. In contrast, a democratic style is one in which a leader encourages all voices to be heard and reaches decisions through consensus. The democratic style may introduce new ideas, share the responsibility to make decisions, and may prove useful in situations in which the leader is uncertain about what path to take, however, it is slow and may also produce decisions that the leader ultimately finds difficult to follow.

A pacesetting leader sets high standards which s/he demonstrates – "do as I do." Although this benchmarking may present an ideal, it may not be attainable by others. One criticism of this style may be, "you became the leader because you were able to do this, now show us an easier way." Followers may be overwhelmed by a pacesetter. As a result, this style works well with highly motivated followers in the short term, but discourages new ideas and responsibility in the longer term. A coaching style of leadership encourages skill development and improvement efforts. It necessitates followers that want to be coached and a leader that knows how to coach.

Most leaders, and most individuals, are most comfortable with one style, but are able to apply and respond to all six styles. An ideal leader would be able to apply a style appropriate to the circumstance, and mix styles as needed. Awareness of one's most comfortable style and conscious use of others may enable a leader to be more effective. In addition, a leader may employ other individuals as a part of his team who use other styles, such that when the two work together, they can produce greater results. Finally, it may be useful to role play prior to an important meeting during which one has to adopt a leadership style that is not as comfortable or not one's usual style.

Managing Physician and Patient Expectations

For physician leaders, managing physicians' expectations can be challenging. In 2012, there were 878,194 licensed physicians in the US, of whom, 75 % were graduates of a US medical school. They are fairly consistently represented in each age category, with 22 % aged 39 years or less, 25 % aged 40–49 years, 24 % aged 50–59 years, 17 % aged 60–69 years, and 9 % aged 70 years old or more (2 % unknown) [9]. Although 66 % of current physicians are male, female physicians represent a greater proportion of entering into practice (8 % versus 2 %).

The majority of physicians in practice today were trained at a time in which care of the individual patient was the focus. Patients were evaluated and treated one at a time, in a face-to-face encounter. Since 1965 or so, reimbursement has been fee-for-service, driven by the service(s) provided and largely paid by employer-based insurance plans, Medicare or Medicaid. Those who trained more than 25 years ago expected to work in solo and independent practice operations and to have open hospital and nursing home staff privileges to allow continuity of care for their patients. Diagnosis and treatment services were largely provided by physicians alone. Specialty referrals were made between physicians at their discretion, between individuals who usually had a professional acquaintance and relationship, with the expected service request implicitly understood. Physicians knew that patients expected a personal relationship with them with relatively easy access. They expected patients to respect their judgment and follow their recommendations. They knew that patients would have little access to their own health information, the medical literature, or other information describing the risks and benefits of various treatments. Patients held little responsibility for the costs invoked in their care, the effect of their personal habits upon their health, or for self-management of disease.

Health care is rapidly moving from a focus on episodic care of the individual patient to preventive and holistic management of a population or panel of patients within a care delivery system that does not always require face-to-face physician contact. Care is often provided by members of a team which may include a variety of physician-extenders, other health care professionals and lay staff, in addition to a physician. Information about disease causation, diagnosis, and treatment is widely available on the internet, and there is a growing emphasis on patient participation in decision-making and patient responsibility in disease management. Rather than purely volume-driven reimbursement for care, the US is moving towards quality or accountability-based metrics for payment. Physicians will largely work in an employment or associated (independent physician association, IPA) model, often within a large multispecialty groups or health systems which provide care across the continuum of sites of service, including ambulatory and acute hospital care, post-acute and home care. Patients and their primary physician may or may not know the providers at other sites in the system. Communication between providers as well as between patients and providers is accomplished via electronic medical records (EMRs), web-based communication and email systems.

Bridging the generational expectations of both physicians and patients is a significant challenge for physician leaders. The average age of licensed physicians in the US is now 51 years. Older physicians have generally valued autonomy, professionalism, beneficence, entrepreneurship and hard work. Younger physicians have demonstrated more comfort with employed models of practice, working in teams, controlled work hours and lifestyle, outcome data-driven decision-making and patient participation in care. In addition, physician leaders also need to navigate changes in expectations regarding physician compensation from a traditional volume-based fee-for-service system to an accountable model based on quality and resource use. In addition, accountable care focuses on the triple aim, improving care for individuals, populations and reducing cost. Expectations surrounding compensation have to incorporate all three aspects of care.

Patient expectations about the provision of medical care and their physicians also vary with age. Older patients have generally maintained their expectation for personal doctor-patient communication rather than electronic access or use of home monitoring methods to communicate and provide clinical data. A diabetic adult may receive care in a "medical home" within an accountable care organization (ACO) where the patient may be assigned a primary care physician, nurse practitioner, diabetic nurse educator, nutritionist and health advocate, and be asked to provide blood sugar assessments through home-based systems. When patients encounter a problem, they may be confused as to whom they should contact. Consideration of the patients' viewpoint when designing systems of care is critical. Physician leaders may employ patients or consumer groups to review protocols or systems prior to implementation as providers may have a "blind spot" for issues that are important to patients. Physician reimbursement may be provided under a managed care mechanism with a per-patient per-month fee or a global fee, which is modified by quality measures (e.g. hemoglobin A1C, the blood pressure, and lipid parameters), in addition to general primary care preventive process measures (e.g. vaccine and cancer screening adherence). Patients may have no knowledge of this incentive arrangement with their physicians.

Why Some Leaders Succeed and Others Fail

Although individuals set their own personal leadership goals and definitions of success or failure, organizations and the individuals being led also assess a leader according to their own values. Success or failure may be defined by achievements, activities, promotions, awards, financial rewards, or recognition. It may be the production of measureable outcomes or qualitative change. It may be enduring or transient. Individuals may succeed as leaders for a variety of reasons – mentoring, timing, technical skill, strategic orientation, personality style, hard work, and/or a partnership with management or others – or they may fail for the very same reasons. They must be successful leaders, who intrinsically understand what is required of them in their leadership roles.

Much has been written about "managing up" – a leader's ability to meet the expectations of a supervisor(s). Physician leaders, in particular, may face a challenge in trying to bridge their clinical acumen with the quality, financial and other results metrics of executive management. They need to shape management's expectations for what can be achieved regarding volume, quality, access, introduction of new techniques and programs, and other outcomes of care such as medical errors and malpractice. They also must bridge their clinical expertise with the financial and other expectations of management who may lack a barometer for clinical outcomes.

Unlike leadership in business or research organizations, however, physician leaders are often still expected to also maintain skills in the practice of medicine – to be a "player-coach." This expectation may have an initial appeal to a new physician leader, allowing him to continue to practice medicine and to show mastery within a familiar area. Depending on the size of the organization and the role, however, the dual roles of clinician and leader may ultimately pose a time management challenge which can lead to failure. The need to grow professionally as a leader requires an investment in time and effort to acquire new knowledge and skills, often occurring at the expense of clinical skills maintained through frequent performance (particularly procedures) and study of the medical literature. The "player-coach" model first described in sports ultimately proved unsustainable in that context, as players were unable to simultaneously perform and coach other players at an outstanding level. It has not been successful in the business arena either [10], yet the "player-coach" model persists in medicine, perhaps due to the strong role identity of a physician. The expectations and proportion of time dedicated to clinical practice – the "player" role – must be carefully managed. For physicians, it may provide credibility, however, it may also derail their leadership role. Most physician leaders still continue to practice in a limited way in order to provide patient contact and the intellectual challenge of medical practice that brought them to the profession. It also provides feedback on the systems that one has developed. Finally, it provides credibility that is often not needed for nonphysician leaders in other discipline or in business. It is likely that physician leaders will pursue medical education first, and then pursue business training during or following clinical training rather than pursuing a business or management degree first as duration of medical training is so long that lessons learned in business training initially may be lost.

Should I Take a Physician Leadership Job?

When considering whether to pursue a physician leadership role, one has to consider many issues. The first should be the importance of different and competing personal goals. A physician may value the impact of his clinical role on patients, the level of interpersonal connection with patients and other physicians, the sense of achievement in performing procedures or in making diagnoses and providing treatment. In contrast, a physician leadership role may attenuate those interpersonal relationships with individual patients and other physicians and limit clinical activity, eroding confidence and skill in practice activities. Nonetheless, the trade-off might be the opportunity to positively impact a larger patient population than in a traditional practice.

Leadership may provide its own intellectual challenges, sense of achievement and interpersonal connection which fulfill these emotional needs. The work of a physician leader should bring a sense of satisfaction and achievement that parallels what a physician feels in the practice and/or teaching of medicine. Leadership roles vary significantly. In some roles, fiscal responsibility, evaluation, hiring and firing of providers is part of the role, may be more stressful, but also more remunerative. Roles involving medical education, clinical processes, quality, and medical direction, may support a larger simultaneous clinical role. Different leaders obtain satisfaction from different roles and responsibilities. One must know one's preferences, strengths, ability to cope with uncertainty and risk. If a physician does not find joy in the practice of medicine, it is uncertain whether moving to a physician leadership position will fill this void as some of the areas of discontent may play a larger unanticipated role in a leadership job. It is also important to try to ascertain whether one will derive pleasure from a medical leadership position, as one does not want to advance to a job that provides less enjoyment. The personal price of providing empathy for patients and families is not mitigated by moving into a physician leadership role; empathy for those being led is always required. Compensation of a physician executive, as compared with clinical practice, is variable, depending on the physician's specialty and hours. While the compensation package is a consideration, it should not be the sole motivation for pursuing a physician leadership role.

Secondly an honest examination of one's personality, strengths and weaknesses should be undertaken to try to identify whether leadership would feel comfortable or pose a challenge to one's personality preferences. This may be undertaken through introspection, use of formal instruments such as the Myers-Briggs test, and feedback from mentors, patient satisfaction reports or 360° evaluations of performance (from direct reports and patients, as well as supervisors). Feedback from interviews, both with prospective employers and executive recruiters provides valuable information as well.

The appeal of increasing responsibility must be weighed against the time, cost, effort and emotional commitment required for professional development, growth and further training, whether it is achieved through formal or "on-the-job" training. Many physician leaders embark on leadership training programs, course work in management and finance, or a formal master's program in business or health care administration. Beware of "the Peter Principle," coined by Laurence J. Peter and Raymond Hull in 1969, who described members of an organization who are initially promoted based on achievement, success, and merit, but who eventually are promoted beyond their level of ability, commonly phrased as, "employees tend to rise to their level of incompetence." One can pursue a leadership position based upon technical expertise in medicine for which you have insufficient competence now or in the future.

Mentorship is critical at each stage of development as a physician, and certainly in academic and leadership roles. A mentor can provide insight about leadership roles, how to pursue these positions, the pleasures and price of leadership, and also identify individual issues in leadership. A mentor is not a coach, as the mentor is often not engaged in the same type of role or present on an ongoing basis. Formal "executive coaching," common in the business world, is increasingly offered to physician leaders. Executive coaching often focuses on change in behavior and/or specific skills, such as public speaking.

Specific Skills for Physician Leaders

John Kotter has commented that "management is about coping with complexity. Leadership, by contrast, is about coping with change" [11]. He describes "the eight stage process of creating major change" which equally applies to health care as it does to business [12]. His steps are: (1) establishing a sense of urgency; (2) creating the guiding coalition; (3) developing a vision and strategy; (4) communicating the change vision; (5) empowering broad-based action; (6) generating short-term wins; (7) consolidating gains and producing more change; and (8) anchoring new approaches to the culture. This stepwise process is applicable to physicians across all roles of leadership. To achieve these stages, physicians must have a set of specific skills which they bring to these steps.

Physician leaders must have or develop a number of skills in their administrative roles beyond their clinical expertise which may include the ability to recruit other physicians; work in and lead teams; negotiate; coordinate care across providers, services, and settings over time; incorporate performance and outcome measurements for improvements and accountability; and perhaps most importantly, adapt to change and bring others with them. Selected areas of skill and knowledge are discussed in the following section. Most of the specific skills described are similar in the administrative and business world, with materials, books, online information and courses available to physician leaders to assist in their development.

Physician Recruitment

Recruitment of physicians and other professional staff is usually the responsibility of physician leaders. An effective leader in physician recruitment tends to have high "emotional intelligence," using the language of Goleman. Several basic skills are required to effectively fulfill this role, including strategic planning and negotiation. Physician leaders need to determine the mix of specialties of physicians required, perform a needs analysis and market assessment, identify the type of relationship between the physicians to be recruited and the organization (employed, contractual, voluntary) and the seniority or level of experience required for the job, develop a job description with supporting staff and equipment, assess applicants, and determine a compensation plan for contractual or employed physicians.

Determining an appropriate mix of providers, primary care and specialists, for a hospital or health system is often influenced by the practice and payment environment, in addition to the needs analysis of the community. The goal in a traditional fee-for-service environment may be to generate and maintain acute care admissions by expanding ambulatory care programs and feeder practices as well as developing high quality acute care services and/or "destination" programs that draw from beyond the local community. In an accountable care organization (ACO) or capitated environment, the goal may be providing enough breath in primary care services to attract, enroll or align patients, while providing sufficient specialty depth both inside and outside of the hospital (the most expensive site of care) to provide required services within the ACO, prevent leakage, and allow for adequate clinical integration such that improvements in quality and savings can occur.

Recruitment objectives may also target services which meet new or growing community needs and/or increase market share, such as the opening of a new pain management program which may be a "loss leader" on its own but may attract new patients and satisfy community needs. Similarly, other recruitment objectives may include the development of programs that improve quality at a lower cost. This same pain management program may also improve quality and reduce overall system costs despite being a loss leader as an individual program. Identification of these opportunities provides an important role in strategic planning for physician leaders.

Thirdly, the model of provider participation for recruitment must also be considered before searching for additional physicians. Is a voluntary or staff model preferred? Or a hybrid? Sometimes the interests of hospitals/health systems diverge from that of the physicians, and a physician leader must be certain whom s/he represents in this leadership role and in recruitment. Examples may include the relationship between voluntary physicians and employed physicians. The hospital may want to maintain voluntary physicians who bring business to their institution without cost and expect that the medical leadership will address the issues of quality, citizenship, length of stay, for example. But in this example, the medical leadership has no leverage to achieve these goals other than providing support and continuing education as a carrot, and recredentialing as the stick, which is very limited as most organizations have an open staff.

Prior to initiation of a search, an institution must perform a needs analysis to develop a job description. This step may seem self-evident, but it is often omitted leading to disappointment later due to differing expectations between a recruit and leadership. For example, a new interventional subspecialist may apply for a position that he/she believes requires only the performance of procedures, while the institution conceives the position to be half procedures and half patient visits. A review of the market and prevalence of disease does not currently support a full time proceduralist.

Leaders must also make initial decisions regarding the required type (specialist, subspecialist, etc.) and level (experience) of expertise required. In an academic setting, the academic rank often identifies the seniority and expertise; however, in the clinical arena, insurance payers do not differentiate between a services provided by a junior or senior physician. Senior or experienced physicians may expect higher compensation than a younger, less experienced physician, but clinical revenues may not allow for it.

The job description may identify the level of specialization, as indicated by procedural skills, board certifications, clinical training and experience, as well as the seniority. For clinical positions, the job description should indicate the volume and types of patients that the prospective physician is expected to manage. If there are quality metrics the physician is expected to achieve, the job description should spell these out, at least in broad terms. For a primary care physician, panel size within an ACO environment and/or quality metrics (process and outcome metrics) should be identified. These may include metrics regarding preventive measures (e.g. vaccines, cancer screening), disease management (blood pressure, hemoglobin A1c, LDL, etc.), and metrics regarding patient communication and office management. For a specialist, volume or work RVU (relative value units) metrics may be included as well as quality metric goals (metrics which are process, disease management and/or communication specific to the specialty). Expectations for clinical, administrative, and/or academic time must be characterized, including committee work, teaching and research, which do not contribute to individual clinical revenues. "On call" or off-hour activity coverage time and compensation must be explicitly described. The level of clinical support and equipment to be provided and any expectations of financial contributions by either party to the cost of support of that staff should be described. These are also areas in which differing expectations often occur. Recruitment and start-up costs can be quite significant, so reaching a clear plan for which party is responsible for the cost of these items, as well as the expected volume or level of activity, is critical.

When developing the job description, explicit plans regarding components and amount of compensation (base salary, incentive plans, contributions to overhead, ownership, etc.), the compensation goal and range, fringe benefits, and other types of compensation (moving support, mortgage assistance, parking, continuing medical education time, tuition assistance, vacation and other personal time, etc.) should be identified prior to beginning a search as these items may represent trades in negotiation with candidates. The manner in which a search is conducted must be also considered. Is the position listed locally, advertised online or with specialty society recruitment materials, or is a recruitment agency to be employed? These agencies may work on a percentage of salary range, on commission or by retainer. A physician leader should be able to identify the expected time frame and cost of a search.

Prior to conducting an interview, the candidate's *curriculum vitae* should be carefully reviewed to identify skills, training, areas of expertise, areas of concern and other topics to engage the candidate in conversation. Missing content, training, time unaccounted for is as informative as the material presented. The care with which a *curriculum vitae* is prepared is often revealing as well. During an interview, it is important to describe the position sufficiently to provide the candidate with an understanding of the role; one must allow sufficient time for the candidate to respond and ask questions of their own. Nonverbal communication should be noted. It is often most difficult to assess clinical competence in the interview, but interpersonal style, flexibility, enthusiasm, energy, motivation, ambition and long term goals should be evident. Ultimately references will be sought to complete the picture of personality as well as clinical competence. It is important to leave the candidate with a positive impression of the institution's leadership as this is a part of building a reputation. There are many resources which provide information about effective interviewing styles and questions which may be useful to leaders new at this role.

Negotiation

Negotiation is a universal skill required by leaders and managers about which much has been written. Negotiations generally fall into two types – distributive (competitive) in which both parties seek to "win," and integrative (cooperative) in which both parties seek an agreement in which both benefit. Apparent distributive negotiations may present internally regarding resources such as funds, space, access, and staff. Although both types of situations present themselves with regularity for physician leaders when working with hospital administration, other departments, recruits or current physician staff, and outside parties, usually such negotiations should become integrative as it is likely that future negotiations with the same party will occur. Externally, negotiations may be increasingly competitive as networks grow and compete for market share. Mergers of systems and "take-overs" of clinical programs, hospitals and medical groups, however, is also occurring and may present opportunities for integrative negotiations as well as both groups identify more opportunities by working together.

Integrative or cooperative negotiations are more creative and useful within an organization as they build relationships and consensus over time between providers, and also with administrative leadership. For example, within an ACO environment, the distribution of shared savings is an example. If shared savings are achieved, how should the money be distributed between primary care and specialists? Should it be based on alignment (primary care physicians brought the patients into the ACO initially) or based upon volume of activity? Or based upon provider's roles in creating the savings by reducing admissions, readmissions and expensive but perhaps unnecessary testing?

Physician recruitment may initially appear to be distributive, as each seeks one's own goals, but should ultimately become integrative, if they are to be successful, as a physician's success may enhance the institution's status, and the tone of the negotiation will influence their ongoing relationship. Distributive negotiations are often a single event in which the two parties part at the end. Integrative negotiations often occur between two parties that must continue to work together after the negotiation is complete.

Preparation for a negotiation is critical. One must learn as much as possible about the issue, identify one's own goals, as well as that of the other party, beforehand. What does each side have that is valuable and can be traded? What do I want? What do they want? What do I have that they want? What can I comfortably give away? How much does reaching an agreement matter to me, or to them? What alternatives to reaching an agreement do we both have? Maintaining an open mind is important; remember "everything is negotiable," although you may decide for yourself what the limits of the negotiation may be. Again, physician recruitment may serve as an example. A physician may want the opportunity to teach, and may accept somewhat lower compensation as a result. On call duty is often a trade in negotiation. It may be included in total compensation or paid as incentive income. Identifying a number of possible trades in schedule, responsibilities, and compensation prior to discussions with candidates may provide a greater chance that the position may be developed in a way that will uniquely appeal to a desired candidate. If both parties are adequately prepared, there is a greater chance of reaching a mutually satisfactory negotiated agreement.

A new leader must ascertain whether there is any history of a prior relationship or hidden issues between the parties as this may color the negotiation. Have any precedents been set between these parties or with similar parties that can influence the outcome of this negotiation? During the negotiation, it is important to "actively listen" as this is a show of good faith. Be cooperative, but "don't let your guard down." Observe body language, emotion as well as verbal and written communication. These signals may not be aligned with the same message. Do not view a smiling, nodding face as someone in agreement; this may just represent active listening by someone who is identifying differences and not reaching a consensus.

Finally, it is important to know when the negotiation is over. It agreement has been reached, how will it be documented and by whom? Is a "sign-off" necessary? By one, or both, parties? Emotional closure is the final step. As Yogi Berra famously said, "it ain't over 'til it's over."

Credentialing and Privileging for Accountable Care

Many physician leaders work within organizations that provides clinical care, whether "bricks and mortar" organizations such as hospitals or clinics, or a virtual ones such as independent physician associations (IPA). The governing boards of such organizations are ultimately responsible for how and what care is provided. Practitioners are largely held responsible for such care, and recruitment, credentialing and privileging of qualified practitioners is an important role for physician leaders. Activities include initial credentialing, re-credentialing, managing and maintaining privileges, and addressing specific provider issues such as: scope of practice (for physicians and other clinicians e.g. nurse practitioners, physician assistants); low or no-volume practitioners; disruptive behavior; decline in physician competence due to aging or medical status; and privileging for novel technologies [13].

Initial credentialing, whether for voluntary or employed practitioners, requires several steps which may be undertaken by the institution (primary source verification) or delegated to a service which provides initial verification data. Some organizations have open medical staffs policy, which allows any individual to apply for clinical privileges, while others require employment or other relationships. These steps include review and verification of data provided in an application for privileges, which, at a minimum, includes education and relevant training sites; board eligibility and certifications; state and special licensure and certifications; drug enforcement agency licensure (DEA); prior and current medical staff positions (voluntary or non-voluntary resignation); malpractice history; clinical experience, current competence and ability; and a background check. Although privileging verification activities are completed by staff, the physician leader is ultimately responsible to review and provide the board with a recommendation regarding the application for privileges.

The physician leader may need to investigate areas of omission of information on an initial application, such as a prior job, training, medical staff membership or malpractice information. Malpractice information must be assessed in the context of years and volume of practice and the nature of the claims. Clinical activity in multiple several states and venues, involuntary resignation of medical staff membership and/or limitation or loss of clinical privileges are areas of concern. The physician leader may find that an interview of the applicant is necessary to reach a decision.

Physician leaders play a particularly important role in defining the specific clinical privileges that providers are granted within the organization and the level of competency that must be demonstrated for each. They "delineate" the privileges, assess the individual, and make a recommendation regarding the individual's request for procedural privileges to the credentialing committee of the Medical Executive Committee, and ultimately, to the governing board. Privileges are often delineated as a detailed checklist or catalog of activities and procedures that a physician may request to perform. Sometimes, particularly for cognitive services, specific privileges may be lumped together as a catalog of specialty-specific "core privileges" which are of low risk clinical activities routinely performed by all individuals in that specialty and are a routine part of training. Other specific privileges may be further characterized by the level of inherent risk to patients and are usually categorized accordingly (level I–III). The privileges which require further expertise may require demonstrated criteria-based competency, in addition to completion of training in that specialty, and/or board certification. This may be accomplished through observation, case logs, record reviews, peer evaluations and other methods, prior to approval.

In 2007 The Joint Commission implemented Focused Professional Practice Evaluation (FPPE) which describes a focused review of a practitioner's activities when a concern is raised about quality, ability or competence for any reason. Planning for a focused practice review must include identification of triggers (including behavioral problems, cognitive and medical changes in providers, competency issues, malpractice, observations and complaints about the quality, attendance, and documentation), scope (which activities), time frame and methodology (chart review, direct observation, data review), who conducts the review and the response to the review.

Most physicians are re-credentialed every 24 months as per the Centers for Medicare and Medicaid Services (CMS) requirement. The Joint Commission expects that the organization has ongoing, objective and outcomes-driven data to support this activity which includes the 2007 Joint Commission requirement of Ongoing Professional Practice Evaluation (OPPE) which is intended to examine all areas of practice rather than specific triggers. For physicians who have no or minimal clinical activity in the organization, so called "low volume" providers (specialists who practice largely in an unassociated ambulatory setting, delegate hospital care to "hospitalists," or perform the majority of patient care at another institution), an ongoing review of care is not possible. Some institutions provide "nonclinical privileges," particularly for physicians participating in administrative or educational activities, or request voluntary resignation of the practitioner in this circumstance.

Physician leaders have a central role in defining the medical staff bylaws regarding credentialing, oversight and review of the process, delineating privileges, performing FPPE and OPPE, and ultimately overseeing credentialing and privileging of practitioners within an organization.

Quality of Care

Quality of healthcare became a national priority with the ground-breaking 2001 Institute of Medicine report, "Crossing the Quality Chasm: a New Health System for the 21st Century." Since that time, there has been a tremendous increase in requirements for hospitals and other healthcare organizations regarding the quality of care, accountability and improvement efforts. These largely emanate from CMS and the Joint Commission (TJC, formerly the Joint Commission on Accreditation of Healthcare Organizations [JCAHO]), a free-standing nonprofit organization that surveys and accredits more than 20,000 healthcare organizations in the United States, as well as from the state. Accreditation by the Joint Commission is often used by the states for licensure and Medicaid reimbursement. CMS requires that organizations maintain effective, ongoing, comprehensive, data-driven quality assessment and performance improvement programs. In addition, National Council on Quality Assurance (NCQA) accreditation for quality and performance is sought by most healthcare organizations.

Definitions of quality, measurement and improvement activities have rapidly escalated since the Affordable Care Act which has focused attention on how to (re)organize the delivery of care to achieve better health system performance, improve outcomes and lower cost. CMS, through the Centers for Medicare and Medicaid Innovation (CMMI) [14], is sponsoring many quasi-experimental delivery and payment programs intended to improve care and reduce costs. Successful improvement and health system reform efforts require stakeholders at all levels to adopt a coherent, systemic approach toward care delivery. Data regarding healthcare system performance and quality has expanded and become publically available [15–17]. CMS has particularly focused on hospital care and readmissions for patients discharged with heart failure, acute myocardial infarction, and pneumonia and imposed financial penalties regarding performance. HEDIS (the Healthcare Effectiveness Data and Information Set) measures are used by more than 90 % of health plans to measure performance on dimensions of care and service. Quality items are now routinely employed in payment schemes for Medicare, Medicaid and commercial managed insurances, for hospitals, nursing homes, and physician practices.

Medicare (CMS) measures fall under "value-based purchasing" domains which are to be implemented over the next several years include [18]: clinical process of care (2013), patient experience of care (2013), outcomes (2014), and efficiency (2015). The patient experience of care domain includes: nurse communication, doctor communication, hospital staff responsiveness, pain management, medicine communication, hospital cleanliness and quietness, discharge information, and overall hospital rating. Clinical processes of care include items related to a diversity of hospital-based clinical care issues. Outcome domain items will include 30-day mortality rates from acute myocardial infarction, heart failure, pneumonia, complications of infections and central line-associated blood stream infection. Efficiency will focus on Medicare spending per beneficiary.

Physician leaders play an essential role in leading quality improvement initiatives which generally focus on patient access, prevention and treatment, costs, safety (including potentially avoidable hospital use), and specific health outcomes. Although credentialing and privileging is a part of this activity, the identification of quality targets, data collection and analysis, and obtaining and determining internal and external benchmarks for clinical activities comprises much of the efforts in quality improvement. The scope of activities must be appropriate to the complexity of the organization, hospital or other healthcare service; involve all areas of activity; focus on improving the quality of care and outcomes of care, while reducing and preventing medical errors (patient safety). Physician leaders may obtain information from the Institute of Medicine's 2013 report, "Toward quality measures for population health and the leading health indicators" and additional training in this area from the Institute for Healthcare Improvement (IHI) and other organizations. While some physician executives may pursue a career specifically in quality improvement, all physician leaders must increasingly be familiar and conversant with quality improvement methodology.

Oversight of Systems of Care and Patient Safety

Physician leaders are often responsible to design and redesign care processes and systems, providing clinical knowledge to identify the population needs within an accountable care system. Choices must be made regarding the process and coordination of care for defined populations within and across a variety of clinical settings. Transitions in care occur when a patient either physically moves from one setting or level of care to another (discharge from hospital to home care, for example) or virtually moves from the care of one physician or team, to another, or both. Within an accountable care environment, patient transitions in care pose the greatest challenge to the integration and smooth delivery of care. Decisions regarding criteria for each component of the system are also required within this new environment in an effort to improve quality while reducing costs. Which patients should have access to intensive care units, for example, and for how long? Who decides? The design of care processes and systems must take into the quality metrics which are reflected in care and payment schemes, patient access and safety, and the strategic plan for the organization.

Physician leaders are also called upon to supervise the provision of care. They must identify what parameters of care to evaluate and what data and information technology infrastructure is required for care assessment, coordination and management. They may use "care managers," "transitional staff" and other professional and nonprofessional staff to assist. Physician leaders must also be engaged in assessing the goals and quality of care provided based upon both their analysis of the evidence in the medical literature, quality parameters imposed by insurance plans, state and federal agencies, as well as institutional priorities.

Patient safety also became a major area of focus for physician leaders since the 1999 publication of the Institute of Medicine report "To Err is Human." In 2005 Patient Safety Organizations (PSOs) were established by law to improve the quality and safety of US health care delivery by encouraging clinicians and health care organizations to voluntarily report and share quality and patient safety information without fear of legal discovery. The Agency for Healthcare Research and Quality (AHRQ) coordinates the development of "Common Formats" for reporting patient safety events to PSOs [19]. Patient safety focuses on medical errors and complications due to systems, practices and culture. When errors occur, they should be comprehensively studied by a patient safety team to alter systems and processes of care to prevent their reoccurrence. Examples are hospital-acquired infections; falls and injury; incorrect administration of a drug, whether associate with dosage, indication, name, or correct patient; iatrogenic hypoglycemia from treatment of diabetes; among others. Physician leaders may be involved in reporting errors, discussions with the team in which they occurred, but also in redesign of processes of care to prevent reoccurrence.

Physician leaders frequently participate in planning direct investments in health care technology. Technology may include electronic medical record and data systems, equipment, and construction. These discussions require information and data linking state-of-the art clinical activities and assessments of current and future needs involving their use, timing of acquisition, cost-benefit analysis and implementation plans. At times, decisions regarding technology made by administration may neglect to consider the time, cost and impact of implementation on clinical practice that physician leaders may anticipate. Although one may not have sufficient knowledge and experience to assess the technology itself, physician leaders are critical to decisions about its use in the processes of care.

Performance Evaluation

Evaluating the performance of physicians, other providers, programs or systems is an important skill for physician leaders. Performance evaluations have become increasingly sophisticated, having evolved from subjective comments and volume-based metrics of clinical activity to a complex system of accountability involving quality metrics, work RVUs, interpersonal abilities, financial parameters, resource use, as well as volume-based metrics and subjective 360° evaluations, among other items. The impact of performance evaluations on behavior is clearly greater when the focus is limited to fewer performance parameters, however, driving performance based upon a few characteristics, such as has been demonstrated in "pay-for-performance" programs, may distort future performance. The old adage, "be careful what you ask for or you just may get it" is applicable here.

Before embarking on establishing a program of performance evaluation, a physician leader must have a sense of the goals, objectives and strategic plan of the medical center, and those for the program and/or individuals being evaluated, to inform and drive performance. Identification of resources available to assist in performance evaluation is critical, including technical data to include clinical, financial, behavioral and market activities; analytical services; and human resources services and support for remediation or other actions that may ensue as a result of performance evaluation.

Initially, the targets or characteristics of performance to be measured must be selected. These targets must be both useful and important (related to goals and objectives), easily obtainable, consistent, and reliable in reflecting clinical performance. In a clinical setting, parameters of volume, quality (both objective and subjective assessments of care) and cost metrics are often used. Secondly, a determination of whether performance should be evaluated at the level of the individual provider, the clinical unit, the specialty, the department or the system, or at several levels must be made. Data may not be obtainable on an individual provider basis, or on an individual patient basis, and performance may be described by parameters for a panel of patients receiving care at one site or by one team.

Selection of the targets for performance and the unit in which it should be measured depends on the goal(s) for performance evaluations; the availability, veracity, timeliness, and ease at which evaluative data can be produced; and the urgency for action. An effort to improve quality, and to reduce costs, emphasized in accountable care, often focuses on the culture of an organization rather than individual performance. The success of accountable care relies upon the degree that clinical integration and group behavior to accrue improved quality and lower costs. Behaviorally driven change of a group may be more difficult to achieve, but may ultimately be more important.

Physicians, however, tend to be more data-driven, thinking-judging (TJ) type personalities as described in the Myers-Briggs Type Indicator, and competitive, responding more to metrics than behaviorally driven change. They may advocate for individual rather than group data, although the latter will assist in improving the activity of "low performers" in their group data through peer pressure. Work RVUs, which reflect the relative level of time, skill, training and intensity required of a physician to provide a given service, is one method for calculating and comparing productive work or effort expended by a physician in treating patients that was popular during the last decade. One may select quality metrics which assess interpersonal skills (HCAPS), procedural performance, and/or the attainment of various clinical parameters characterizing a panel of patients or a process of care (value-based purchasing parameters, etc.). Once targets are chosen, issues of measurement and benchmarking methodology, frequency and interval, sample, and ultimately, how to communicate and use the data to drive performance change are equally important. Too often excessively detailed data is provided to leaders who do not have time to digest and act upon it, or data is not timely, useful, or is too variable to be useful. Metrics which may be used at the physician level in performance evaluation may include work RVUs, quality metrics, and within academic medical centers, teaching evaluations and scholarly activity, however group quality measures, cost and savings measures, and volume data are the future although the data management may still present a challenge.

Some physician leaders perform yearly appraisals of physicians' performance including clinical, administrative, personal, and in academic medical centers, teaching and scholarly activity. This appraisal may have an impact on compensation, job role, academic promotion, and may provide a concrete vehicle for feedback to the clinician. A leader may need to use any one or all of the leadership styles discussed previously in order to try to support but also drive the physician's behavior and activities in one direction or another. The components of emotional intelligence are critical to success in these meetings – the leader's ability to listen, empathize, appraise, provide feedback and control his own behavior regarding the physician's responses – as well as some brief preparation prior to these meetings and follow up afterwards.

Preparation for communicating a physician's performance evaluation is important. One technique is to provide individual performance data with either internal or external benchmarks for comparison prior to the meeting. It may be useful to have the physician complete and submit a self-assessment prior to the meeting. This may include a listing of key result areas, achievements, time utilization, and support required to improve performance, as well as desired areas and longer term career planning. The conduct of the meeting is important. Is the physician seated next to the leader or across the desk? As with patient interviews, it is most helpful to start with open-ended subjective comments, such as "how do you think you are doing?" before narrowing the discussion to the particular issues and data. It is critical to have a common understanding of what is expected of the physician and whether he has the resources to achieve these goals.

Areas which may be included in physician performance evaluations include:

Clinical activities:

- Clinical knowledge – board certifications, other measures
- Professional competence/quality of care – procedural data or clinical (blood pressure control, hemoglobin A1C, vaccination rates, etc.)
- Patient experience (satisfaction) data
- Productivity data – volume, wRVUs, etc.
- Resource utilization (depends on specialty)
- Peer and staff relationships (a 360° evaluation is performed)

Educational activities:

- Teaching hours and content and trainees
- Teaching evaluations
- Teaching curricula, participation in national educational committees and programs

Research (basic or clinical):

- Status of current projects, mentoring
- Grants submitted, funded, status
- Presentations and publications
- Professional recognition

Administrative:

- Committee participation (role, hours)
- Contributions to the organization and community
- Administrative role evaluation

Personal:

- Work habits
- Current career goals and plan for the next year
- Five year goals and plan
- Compensation

If the leader intends to use the meeting for feedback, it is important to provide positive feedback before critical comments, and then conclude again with the positive comments, using the "feedback sandwich" method. Following this performance evaluation, it is important to document the findings and the discussion, and provide a copy to the physician, indicating that "I believe that I have captured our discussion herein, but I wanted to provide you with another opportunity to comment if I have not." This serves several purposes. As with patients, employees may stop listening at some point during the discussion, have understood something completely different, or deny that certain content was discussed. The "memo to file" serves to reinforce the discussion points and can be referred to in the future. If the meeting is intended to provide praise only or is a retention meeting, the document further reinforces the leader's enthusiasm for this individual. It may be useful to have the individual acknowledge receipt if the memo is to be kept as part of an employment or compensation issue.

Physician leaders are often charged with driving physician performance as a part of institutional efforts to drive performance. Employee engagement describes the enthusiasm and avidity, both emotionally and intellectually, with which employees approach and fulfill their jobs. The literature describes a number of important drivers of employee engagement in the business world which retain some validity in the health care environment [20]:

- Trust and integrity (of managers)
- Nature of the job – is it mentally stimulating day-to-day?
- Line of sight between employee and company performance
- Career growth opportunities
- Pride about the company
- Coworkers/team members
- Employee development
- Personal relationship with one's manager

Examples of specific efforts to increase employee engagement in healthcare organizations may focus broadly or specifically depending on the goal [21].

Financial and Legal Skills for Physician Leaders

Physician leaders need a basic level of familiarity with legal issues which may include knowledge of employment law, malpractice, and antifraud laws. Employment law pertains to hiring, firing, harassment, state licensure rules, immigration law, scope and ability to practice (physical/psychological) as well as other issues within a medical program. Discussions of wages and compensation, labor standards and productivity, rules pertaining to full-time versus part-time and per diem employment, union versus non-union employees, and the use of physician extenders and paraprofessionals are some of the employment law issues. In addition, management of physician impairment and behavior may invoke a variety of legal issues. Partnership with human resource and legal counsel is highly recommended and often required because it is often unfamiliar to new physician leaders who may have functioned as independent entities in their own practices outside of the compliance regulations and medical staff bylaws. But across many healthcare institutions, particularly those participating in ACO collaborations, employment models are increasingly popular as they provide additional levers of control for organizations to encourage physician behavior with regard to quality metrics.

Familiarity with antifraud issues regarding clinical care and insurance, incentives regarding quality-focused programs in medical care, Stark law against self-referral and anti-kickback schemes are also particularly important in accountable care organizations as well as fee-for-service arrangements. The Stark law limits physician referrals, prohibiting referrals for health services for patients insured by Medicare or Medicaid to an entity in which the physician (or family member) has a financial relationship. For example, a physician cannot refer patients in his practice to a laboratory, radiology service, physical therapy or hospital for testing or treatment in which he is an owner-operator.

Financial skills for physician leaders may range from budgeting, designing compensation arrangements, to negotiating acquisitions of clinical equipment and facilities and practices. Familiarity and some facility with basic accounting principles including the concepts of assets, liabilities, and equity are useful. The ability to understand key financial statements, including balance sheets, income statements, statements of cash flows and cash versus accrual accounting, is also helpful. Although budgets are usually prepared by others, it is essential that physician leaders understand the basic data informing the budget and the type of budget. Physician leaders should be able to use Excel spreadsheet programs, pivot tables, and simple budgeting and statistical elements in these computer programs, as well as how to create a simple budget (income and expense categories) and a basic business plan. These skills can be learned through mini-course formats from physician executive organizations, business school courses and "on-line" courses and materials.

Some examples of clinical (nonacademic) physician leadership roles, job description items are listed in Table 3.1, although these are not all inclusive. As these roles vary across healthcare organizations, so do some of these responsibilities, which may appear within different roles. This list is partial but may provide descriptive content.

Table 3.1 Job descriptions for physician leadership roles

Roles	Chief medical officer	Medical director	Chairman, medical staff	Clinical team or facility directors or service line directors	Director of quality	Director of care or case management (although care and case management are not synonymous, they are often used interchangeably)
	Hospital, Health System or Health Plan, ACO	Hospital, unit, ambulatory facility, long term care facility, home care agency, insurance entity, subsection of any of the prior mentioned, or insurance, vendor or pharmaceutical entity	Hospital, health system, multispecialty ambulatory network or group			
Regulatory compliance	Establish and oversee compliance with all medical policies, directives, rules, regulations and clinical performance standards of the state, federal government, hospital bylaws and accrediting bodies. Oversee and manage all on-site inspections, assisting inspectors and surveyors in the performance of their duties, and provides reports as required to follow-up	Collaborate with the organization's senior leadership to ensure medical compliance with all customer, regulatory, and accreditation requirements for clinical services; develop strong compliance and accreditation programs	Support and encourage regulatory compliance among medical staff	Support and encourage regulatory compliance among medical staff. Direct quality evaluation and improvement and reporting on health and quality assurance issues	Collect, analyze, and report data regarding patient care. Interface Assess and report quality metrics required by accreditation agencies, federal, state, local, and health plans as well as internally chosen metrics, to ensure compliance with rules and regulations and specifications	

(continued)

Table 3.1 (continued)

Policies and procedures	Assure the ongoing development and implementation of policies and procedures *that guide and support the provision of medical staff services*	Develop policies and procedures and provide guidance and medical leadership and direction for *clinical* policies, procedures	Review and comment upon policies and procedures	Develop policies and procedures and provide guidance and medical leadership and direction for *clinical* policies, procedures	Develop policies and procedures regarding quality – for example, infection control, perioperative care, etc.	
Credentialing and clinical authority	Ensure appointment of medical staff and allied health privileges are compliant with sound credentialing practices. Act as the organization's ultimate authority on medical issues		Establish and oversees credentialing and privileging activities			
Leadership role	Perform as an effective leader regarding skills of delegation, organization, and coordination for intra-department activities and inter-department integration	Function as a role model and establish authority but shared responsibility regarding ethics, clinical practice and quality with providers	Function as a role model and establish authority but shared responsibility regarding ethics, clinical practice and quality with providers	Arrange and conducts regular meetings of clinical providers, conduct team management and performance evaluation and improvement	Represent the organization at departmental, organizational, community or business meetings regarding existing or proposed clinical services	Maintain knowledge of current and emerging information regarding clinical care, insurance coverage, quality metrics and payment plans and legislative requirements regarding care and/or case management services

External representation	Represent the institution in community organization activities designed to modify community behavior, epidemiology, and/or needs	Provide physician relations or representation to community and outside organizations	Provide physician relations or representation to the community and outside organizations		Collaborate with community-based programs, nongovernmental agencies and social services and health care organizations to address patient needs and or barriers to improved health outcomes
Finance	Assist in the development and presentation of the clinical activities budget, including staffing, support plan, and equipment needs projections	Evaluate clinical performance		Evaluate and report clinical and financial metrics regarding group performance	Participate in discussions and problem solving for key variances and outcomes identified related to areas of direct responsibility which have fiscal impact

(continued)

Table 3.1 (continued)

Clinical operations	Develop the organizational plan for clinical operations and provide for efficient use of personnel. Assess and communicate recommendations for utilization of space, space needs, equipment, personnel and other resources as needed	Provide leadership and guidance on clinical programs; monitor and improve quality and appropriateness of medical care, implement clinical practice guidelines and/or best practices based on evidence, lead peer review activities; oversee/develop provider education and training activities. Manage clinical operations within the clinical unit; work with nursing and administrative leadership to achieve high efficiency and quality in clinical operations. Review patient satisfaction survey; function as first-level patient complaint solution focal point. Lead or participates in review of practice management functions, e.g., reception, telephone triage, patient flow, outreach services, laboratory, follow-up on missed appointments, referral tracking, etc.	Provide leadership and guidance on clinical programs; monitor and improve quality and appropriateness of medical care, implement clinical practice guidelines and/or best practices based on evidence, lead peer review activities; oversee/develop provider education and training activities. Manage clinical operations within the clinical unit; work with nursing and administrative leadership to achieve high efficiency and quality in clinical operations. Review patient satisfaction survey; function as first-level patient complaint solution focal point. Lead or participates in review of practice management functions, e.g., reception, telephone triage, patient flow, outreach services, laboratory, follow-up on missed appointments, referral tracking, etc.	Develop system or institution-wide quality initiatives and assist with roll-out to clinical units. Leads review of procedures related to quality and process improvement activities, studies and programs Develop, monitor and report on analytical and statistical reports of performance metrics and operations. Oversees utilization management	Create an effective and efficient design and delivery of care management programs, services and staffing to accomplish established operational and financial objectives. Lead programs regarding care management and pharmacy utilization, transitions programs, discharge services across the continuum of care. Serve as a liaison to the Primary Care Providers as questions arise regarding care managers or care management protocols

Personnel	Prepare and recommends qualifications statements for credentialing, job descriptions, and evaluation standards for all clinical personnel. Develop an effective process for staff development and retention	Responsible for clinical assignments, rotation and call schedules, coverage and approval of leave time, etc.		Responsible for clinical assignments, rotation and call schedules, coverage and approval of leave time, etc.	Develop a program of excellence to insure interdisciplinary teams are utilizing state-of-the art best practices for preventative care, clinical care delivery and coordination and population management. Effectively work with clinical teams to meet patient outcome measures and performance goals defined by the strategic plan. Serve as a clinical leader and resource for care managers and care management staff
Medical information technology	Advise on health information system, technology and equipment needs; develops, recommends, and conducts special studies of health needs and priorities, interprets clinical data	Advise and implement electronic medical records systems and enforce Meaningful Use (MU)		Assist in quality data collection through use of electronic medical records	Use data to drive decisions and plan/implement performance improvement strategies related to care management for patients assigned to staff to include fiscal, clinical and patient satisfaction data

(continued)

Table 3.1 (continued)

Strategic planning	Provide clinical leadership for strategic planning, strategy execution and implementation of clinical and care management programs	Participate in strategic planning and program development		Identify opportunities for new program development to achieve quality improvement

References

1. Kruze K. What is leadership. Forbes Mag. 2013. Available at: http://www.forbes.com/sites/kevinkruse/2013/04/09/what-is-leadership/Forbes. Accessed 16 Aug 2013.
2. Goleman D. What makes a leader? Harvard Business Review on what makes a leader. Boston: Harvard Business School Publishing Corporation; 1998–2001. p. 1–26.
3. Myers Briggs Personality Inventory ®. 2013. Available at: http://www.personalitydesk.com/product/myers-briggs-type-indicator-online?gclid=CKHCgsbj8bgCFcef4AodMh0AhA. Accessed 9 Aug 2013.
4. Zardouz S, German MA, Wu EC, Djalilian HR. Personality types of otolaryngology resident applicants as described by the Myers-Briggs Type Indicator. Otolaryngol Head Neck Surg. 2011;144(5):714–8.
5. Swanson JA, Antonoff MB, D'Cunha J, Maddaus MA. Personality profiling of the modern surgical trainee: insights into generation X. J Surg Educ. 2010;67(6):417–20.
6. Aranda R, Tlton S. Myers-Briggs personality preferences may enhance physician leadership success in non-clinical jobs. PEJ. 2013;39:14–20.
7. Gorman J. Eight lessons for up-and-coming execs. Wharton leadership lecture. Whart Mag. 12 May 2012. Available at: http://whartonmagazine.com/blogs/james-gormans-eight-lessons-for-up-and-coming-execs. Accessed 9 Aug 2013.
8. Goleman D. Leadership that gets results. Harv Bus Rev. 2000; March–April:82–83.
9. Young A, Chaudhry HJ, Thomas JV, Dugan M. Census of actively licensed physicians in the United States, 2012 Federation of State Medical Boards. J Med Regul. 2013;99(2):11–24.
10. The Boston Consulting Group, Inc. The fallacy of the player-coach model. 2006. Available at: http://www.bcg.com.cn/export/sites/default/en/files/publications/articles_pdf/Fallacy_of_the_Player-Coach_Model_Apr06.pdf. Accessed 9 Aug 2013.
11. Kotter JP. What leaders really do. Harv Bus Rev. December 2001. Available at: http://hbr.org/2001/12/what-leaders-really-do/ar/1. Accessed 21 Oct 2013.
12. Kotter JP. Leading change. Boston: Harvard Business School Press; 1996.
13. Safeek YM. Credentialling & privileging for accountable care. Am Coll Phys Execut. 2012.
14. http://innovation.cms.gov/
15. The Commonwealth Fund Commission on a High Performance Health System. Rising to the challenge: results from a scorecard on local health system performance. New York: Commonwealth Fund; 2012.
16. http://www.hospitalcompare.hhs.gov and http://www.medicare.gov/nursinghomecompare/search.html?AspxAutoDetectCookieSupport=1
17. http://www.health.ny.gov/press/releases/2009/2009-07-24_angioplasty_and_cardiac_surgery_reports.htm
18. http://www.cms.gov/Outreach-and-Education/Medicare-Learning-Network-MLN/MLNProducts/downloads/Hospital_VBPurchasing_Fact_Sheet_ICN907664.pdf. Accessed 22 Aug 2013.
19. http://www.pso.ahrq.gov/formats/commonfmt.htm
20. Gibbons J. Employee engagement: a review of current research and its implications. Research report of the Conference Board, New York; 2006. p. 5. Available at http://montrealoffice.wikispaces.com/file/view/Employee+Engagement+-+Conference+Board.pdf. Accessed 21 Aug 2013.
21. Patrnchak JM. Building an engaged workforce at Cleveland Clinic. J Healthc Leadersh. 2013;5:9–20.

Chapter 4
The ABCs of ACOs

Hope Glassberg, Anne Meara, Carolyn S. Blaum, and Laurie G. Jacobs

> *A straight line may be the shortest distance between two points, but it is by no means the most interesting.*
>
> – Doctor Who

Abbreviations

ACA	Affordable Care Act
ACO	Accountable Care Organization
AMA	American Medical Association
BBA	Balanced Budget Act
CMMI	Centers for Medicare and Medicaid Innovations
CMS	Centers for Medicare and Medicaid
E&M	Evaluation and Management [Codes]
ESRD	End Stage Renal Disease

H. Glassberg • A. Meara, BSN, MBA
Care Management Organization, Montefiore Medical Center,
200 Corporate Boulevard, Yonkers, NY 10701, USA
e-mail: hglassbe@montefiore.org; ameara@montefiore.org; ameara6137@aol.com

C.S. Blaum, M.D., MS
Department of Medicine, Division of Geriatric Medicine and Palliative Care,
NYU School of Medicine, NYU Langone Medical Center,
530 First Avenue, BCD612, New York, NY 10016, USA
e-mail: Caroline.Blaum@nyumc.org

L.G. Jacobs, M.D. (✉)
Department of Medicine, Montefiore Medical Center and Albert Einstein
College of Medicine, 111 East 210 Street, Bronx, NY 10467, USA
e-mail: lajacobs@montefiore.org

© Springer International Publishing Switzerland 2015
J.S. Powers (ed.), *Healthcare Changes and the Affordable Care Act*,
DOI 10.1007/978-3-319-09510-3_4

FFS	Fee-for-Service
FQHC	Federally Qualified Health Center
HHS	Health and Human Services
HMO	Health Maintenance Organization
IPA	Independent Practice Association
MedPAC	Medicare Payment Advisory Commission
MMA	Medicare Modernization Act
MSSP	Medicare Shared Savings Program
NPRM	Notice of Proposed Rulemaking
PGP	Physician Group Practice demonstration
PPO	Preferred Provider Organization
PSO	Provider Sponsored Organization
SGR	Sustainable Growth Rate
TIN	Tax Identification Number

Introduction

The Affordable Care Act substantially raised the national profile of a new healthcare delivery system financing model called accountable care organizations (ACOs). Put very simply, ACOs are groups of healthcare providers that join together and agree to be financially and clinically accountable for patients who seek most of their care from them. While the ACO is considered a relatively new approach, its origins can be traced back to a much earlier period in American healthcare history.

Brief History of the Medicare Program

By the early 1950s in the United States, several attempts to institute a major national health insurance program had surfaced and fizzled. Significant health insurance proposals had emerged under the Theodore Roosevelt, Franklin Roosevelt, and Harry Truman presidencies, but partisan fighting and consistent opposition from the American Medical Association, which viewed the nascent efforts as "socialistic" and financially detrimental to physicians, ultimately stymied efforts [1].

By the 1950s however, the political climate was ripe for consideration of a more limited national insurance program restricted to the elderly – a group widely accepted to be underinsured and burdened by poverty and sickness. At that time, almost half of the elderly population in the United States lacked health insurance [2]. To make the proposal more palatable, proponents initially suggested that the insurance program cover only hospitalization services [1].

After years of political maneuvering and interim steps on the path to a national program, in 1964, supporters of a federal Medicare program had secured both the presidency and a majority in the House and Senate; this advantageous political climate enabled program supporters to propose a more far-reaching program than one restricted to hospitalization only. The resulting Social Security Act amendments in 1965 included a so-called "three layer cake" [3] of programs. One layer "Part A," consisted of coverage for hospitalization; another layer, "Part B" was a voluntary program that required beneficiaries to pay premiums in return for coverage of physician visits; and the last layer, a joint federal-state initiative focused on the poor, would become the Medicaid program [1].

Medicare FFS Versus Managed Care History and Payment Mechanics

At its inception, Medicare was predominantly a "fee-for-service" (FFS) program, meaning that the federal government would pay a fee to healthcare providers for each service rendered. In the Part A program, institutions were paid based upon the costs they incurred and in the Part B program, physicians were paid "allowed charges," defined as the customary, prevailing charge for such services [4].

Some decades earlier, an alternative to FFS medicine had emerged, primarily for employed populations: the concept of prepaid health plans, an early type of managed care plan. During the Great Depression, several doctors – Drs. Michael Shadid, Donald Roos, H. Clifford Loos, and Sidney Garfield – had all developed subscription like models in their respective geographies through which workers and their families would pay the doctors a set monthly fee in return for medical care, when needed [5]. Ultimately, individual fiefdoms of doctors banded together to create entire pre-paid networks of medical providers, the early prototype of what would become Health Maintenance Organizations (HMO). Famous group practices that launched such pre-paid plans included Kaiser Permanente in California, Group Health Association in Washington D.C., Group Health Cooperative in Washington state, and the Health Insurance Plan of New York. In these cases, the entity managing healthcare finances was also responsible for actually delivering clinical care [1].

While these plans were able to enroll sizable numbers of beneficiaries in relatively confined geographic areas, medical societies, including the American Medical Association (AMA), prevented widespread adoption of such plans, expressing concerns that business staff would interfere with medical practice and that medical professionals taking on business responsibilities would engage in improper contracting practices [5]. Consequently, when the Medicare program was established, the notion of managed care was still relatively limited; in the early 1970s there were under 50 HMOs nationally [6].

Managed care in the Medicare program expanded in the 1970s, when the government implemented demonstration programs that provided prepayments to HMOs, organizations responsible for operating networks of providers available to deliver a comprehensive set of medical services to beneficiaries [7]. Much like any other kind of budget, prepayments set a financial ceiling and then deferred to plans and providers to determine an appropriate allocation of funds underneath that ceiling. The prepayments provided the benefit of allowing the government to proactively budget for patient healthcare costs, instead of waiting for costs to accrue on a FFS basis. The prepayment demonstrations also coincided with a broad national effort to expand HMOs–the HMO Act of 1973, which provided $375 million in funds to support the expansion of HMOs, through grants, contracts, and loans. The Act also required employers to provide an HMO option to employees [8].

By the mid-1980s, the Medicare risk based contracting demonstrations became a permanent fixture of the Medicare program, in part due to a growing body of research indicating that HMOs reduced healthcare costs [7]. A famous randomized controlled trial that compared participants in the Group Health Cooperative of Puget Sound, one of the early prepaid physician groups, to individuals seeking care FFS found seemingly impressive impacts –the expenditure rate for all healthcare services was 25 % less among those receiving services from the Cooperative compared to the FFS group [9]. Of note, patients enrolled in the HMO product were less satisfied than their FFS counterparts, perhaps signifying that individuals highly valued the unrestricted FFS provider networks [7].

Cost Pressures and Medicare Managed Care Expansion and Contraction

Over time, managed care became a conceptually bigger part of the Medicare program, particularly as cost pressures became more acute. Post 1965, the cost of the Medicare program far exceeded any predictions. There were several reasons for the outsized cost growth including an initial pent-up-demand for healthcare among the elderly who gained coverage under Medicare; a Part A payment structure that encouraged hospitals to provide a high volume of services; and the fact that increases in beneficiary payments (premiums) paid to the Part B program were tied to inflation and yet Part B cost growth far exceeded inflation growth [2]. By the mid 1990s, Medicare's share of the federal budget had more than doubled since the program began and was the third largest component of the federal budget [10].

Policymakers initiated several major payment reforms to mitigate cost growth, such as the inpatient prospective payment system and the physician fee schedule, both of which set out to bring order to Part A and B payment policies and reduce incentives to inappropriately increase volume of service use among beneficiaries [7]. Another increasingly attractive cost containment tool was managed care.

HMOs were appealing because of studies like the one described earlier that suggested that HMOs could deliver care more efficiently, at lower cost. Reflecting this belief, initially prepayments to HMO plans (also called capitated payments) were pegged to 95 % of the average FFS Medicare costs in the county where the plan was operating [11]. In setting the payment rate at 95 % of the expected FFS costs in a given county, policymakers thought they would be preemptively achieve cost reductions.

The Balanced Budget Act of 1997 (BBA) entrenched the presence of HMOs and other types of managed care plans in the Medicare program even further, formally establishing the Medicare Part C program, known as Medicare Advantage today [12]. Beneficiaries could elect to enroll in a managed care plan, Part C, or remain in traditional FFS Medicare, Parts A and B. In addition to HMOs, the BBA allowed the Medicare program to include a number of other types of managed care plans that had proliferated in the private market and offered various types of networks and approaches for managing utilization of healthcare services.

At the same time as attempting to expand the program, policymakers also sought to right-size payments to managed care plans. Despite best efforts to build cost reductions into capitated payments, in practice, HMOs did not reduce costs. Initially, Medicare HMO payments were tied to average FFS costs incurred by beneficiaries, both healthy and sick, in a given county. The payments assumed that HMO plans would enroll an average cross section of beneficiaries, both healthy and sick. But to the extent that HMO plans enrolled a relatively healthy population, they would essentially be overpaid because the underlying payment reflected costs associated with some sicker beneficiaries. This scenario is exactly what happened– sicker beneficiaries tended to remain in Medicare FFS, while healthier beneficiaries enrolled in managed care; some estimates suggested that the government overpaid managed care plans by as much as $2 billion [13].

The BBA attempted to reign in some of this inappropriate spending by limiting payment increases in geographic areas with relatively high HMO prepayments [7]. Facing this reduction, a number of managed care companies withdrew from markets entirely, thereby involuntarily dis-enrolling sizable numbers of patients. In other cases, to make the new economics work, Medicare managed care plans curtailed benefits available to beneficiaries, reduced payments to providers, or instituted additional steps before beneficiaries could access care, like requiring primary care providers to serve as "gatekeepers," to specialty care. Practices like these, which were widespread in the private market as well, resulted in a significant public backlash against managed care [14]. By the early 2000s, 12 % of Medicare beneficiaries were enrolled in managed care plans instead of FFS; the managed care enrollment rate had actually declined since the passage of the BBA [7].

Subsequent legislation, like the 2003 Medicare Modernization Act (MMA), increased payments to Medicare managed care plans to revive the role of private plans in Medicare and alleviate the cost pressures that had precipitated the earlier backlash. Enrollment in Medicare managed care did in fact rise after its passage, tripling between 2004 and 2013 [11]. In adjusting the payment to plans, however, the MMA further eroded the short-term prospect of managed care as a cost containment tool in the Medicare program. One analysis found that Medicare spent an additional $922 on average for Medicare managed care enrollees compared to comparable beneficiaries in Medicare FFS, leading to extra payments in excess of $5.2 billion by 2005 [15].

Provider-Based Accountability: A Throwback

By the early 2000s, the viability of managed care as a cure-all for reducing Medicare expenditures had diminished, but the cost pressures facing the Medicare program had not eased. In addition, despite the growth of managed care plan enrollment after the MMA's passage, the majority of Medicare beneficiaries were not enrolled in health plans, but rather remained in the program's traditional FFS program. Seeking to experiment with non-HMO/managed care models to reduce costs and improve quality in the FFS context, in 2005, the Centers for Medicare and Medicaid Services launched the Physician Group Practice (PGP) demonstration.

This demonstration allowed ten large physician group practices, six of which were multi-specialty practices and one of which was a physician-hospital organization [16], with at least 200 participating providers to access savings relative to a pre-determined spending benchmark associated with Medicare FFS beneficiaries who sought care from their providers. Savings were also tied to provider performance on 32 quality metrics [16].

> **Sidebar: PGP Demonstration Outcomes**
> The PGP demonstration ran from 2005 to 2010, with a 2-year extension after 2010. Results from the demonstration were positive from a quality perspective – all of the participating ten groups met nearly all of the quality metrics (29 out of 32 metrics) – but the financial outcomes were more modest. In order to access shared savings, demonstration participants had to both meet quality outcomes and achieve a minimum savings rate of 2 %. Half of the demonstration participants saved more than 2 % more than halfway into the demonstration [17, 18].

Around the same time as the PGP demonstration, the term "accountable care organization" began to enter the healthcare lexicon. One of the first explicit national discussions of an ACO model emerged at a November 2006 meeting of the Medicare Payment Advisory Commission (MedPAC), an independent congressional agency tasked with advising Congress about issues pertaining to the Medicare program. MedPAC had been directed by Congress to examine alternatives to the Sustainable Growth Rate (SGR) system, which was intended to adjust physician payments on the basis of changes in input prices, growth in Medicare FFS enrollment, and increases in physician service volume compared to national economic experience [19]. Over time, the SGR system had created a system that dictated physician fee cuts that in the words of one expert, far "exceed[ed] the magnitude of the willingness to cut fees" [19]. During the meeting, Dr. Elliott Fisher, Professor of Medicine at Dartmouth Medical School, surmised that part of the solution would involve an attempt to "strengthen local organizational accountability for the decisions that drive higher costs and worse quality [20]."

Dr. Fisher outlined a process for creating virtual organizational structures (as opposed to established physician groups – the basic organizational unit in the PGP demonstration) to take on financial and clinical accountability; he suggested that such organizations were important because small groups of providers could not significantly influence cost and quality outcomes and that there were relatively few large multispecialty practices in the United States. To create such structures of providers – "extended hospital staff" – he commented that nearly all physicians could be attributed to a hospital either by virtue of being employed by the hospital or because a majority of the patients the physician saw were admitted to a particular hospital when seeking inpatient services.

Second, most beneficiaries could be assigned to a "predominant care physician," either a primary care provider or a specialist that accounted for most of the care they would receive in a given time period. Because of these linkages, he argued, medical groups consisting of diverse arrays of physicians and an anchoring hospital, could reasonably be held accountable for the cost and quality outcomes associated with attributed beneficiaries [20].

By first creating loose organizational structures, borne out of imputed physician relationships to particular hospitals and beneficiary ties to those providers, Dr. Fisher and other meeting participants moved the national dialogue closer to the current incarnation of accountable care organizations. In many ways, by conferring financial and clinical responsibility upon a single organization, the ACO model resembled the early pre-paid physician group practices and HMOs, without the network limitation features that had led to a managed care criticisms in the 1990s [21].

The Affordable Care Act and ACOs

Nearly 300 pages into the Affordable Care Act text, drafters picked up the thread from the PGP demonstration and the MedPAC discussion in a section titled "Encouraging Development of New Patient Care Models." While the provisions in this section generated less public attention – and controversy – in the lead up to the law's passage than provisions pertaining to the health insurance exchanges, collectively, its implications were arguably just as sweeping [22].

Section 3021 of this portion of the act established a Center for Medicare and Medicaid Innovation (CMMI) to experiment with innovative payment and service delivery models focused on reducing Medicare and Medicaid program expenditures, while preserving or ideally enhancing the quality of care provided to beneficiaries. The guiding principle behind CMMI's initiatives is a framework known as the triple aim. The triple aim, developed by the Institute for Healthcare Improvement, a Massachusetts-based non-profit dedicated to advancing health care systems throughout the world, includes the following tenets [23]:

- Improving the patient experience (including quality and satisfaction)
- Improving the health of populations
- Reducing per capita cost of health care

In IHI's formulation, these three aims collectively maximize the performance of health systems: The Act appropriated no less than $10 billion dollars [24] between fiscal years 2011 and 2019 for the fledgling center to meet this call to action.

The Act also enumerated the center's portfolio of activities, which included the promulgation of accountable care organization (ACO) models. In the Act's formulation, outlined in section 3022, Medicare Shared Savings Program (MSSP) ACOs would be comprised of various groups of providers with shared governance structures; that would be "willing to become accountable for the quality, cost, and overall care of the Medicare FFS beneficiaries" assigned to these groups. The Act also held open the possibility for the Secretary of Health and Human Services (HHS) to test a novel variation on the MSSP that would enable highly integrated delivery systems, rather than health insurance companies, to take on partial capitation [22]. While the law delineated the broad financial parameters of the program, it did not go into great depth about how the program would be operationalized or clinical expectations.

Detail arrived a little over a year later when the Centers for Medicare and Medicaid Services released what is known as a (NPRM) codifying section 3022 of the law [25]. Once Congress enacts laws, federal agencies, like the U.S. Department of Health and Human Services, derive authority from the enacted law to issue regulations that detail how the agency intends to implement its provisions [26]. Before regulations are finalized, agencies must seek public input on a proposed version of the regulation [27].

CMS issued its proposed rule on ACOs in April of 2011 [25]. Among other areas, the NPRM sought public input on the idea of creating two ACO options, so as to encourage the broadest possible range of provider groups to participate. Option one, the MSSP, included a one-sided model through which groups of providers that sufficiently managed beneficiaries' expenditures underneath a pre-determined threshold could share in those savings. The model was considered one-sided because participating providers could only gain financially or, at worst, remain neutral, but they would not bear any financial losses as a result of the program [25].

Capitalizing on language in the ACA enabling the Secretary of HHS to test a variation of MSSP, the NPRM also detailed specifics of a "two-sided model" that HHS would offer, called a Pioneer ACO, that would allow organizations with more experience managing financial risk to take a bigger cut of any savings reaped, but also to be accountable for a portion of losses, if incurred [25]. The second option was geared toward systems that already had years of experience taking on financial risk [28].

By early 2012, the two programs had officially launched, with the Pioneer ACO program beginning in January 2012 and the MSSP program starting in April 2012 [29]. Several of the physician groups that had participated in the PGP demonstration elected to participate in a transitional program that aligned with MSSP parameters or the Pioneer ACO program [30]. ACOs were no longer mythic "unicorns" as some healthcare commentators had jokingly termed the much talked about but yet to be implemented model [31]. The text below outlines key features of the two programs.

Key Features of Medicare Pioneer and MSSP ACO Programs

Provider Participation and Length of Programs

Groups of healthcare providers and hospital systems can join together to form a Medicare ACO. Critically, participants in either the MSSP or Pioneer program must have a Medicare-enrolled Tax identification number (TIN); ACOs may comprise a single TIN or multiple TINs [32]. Specifically, physician group practices, provider group organizations (PPOs), independent physician associations (IPAs), employed staff in medical organizations, joint ventures between hospitals and physician organizations, as well as some critical access hospitals, rural health clinics, and federally qualified health centers (FQHCs), can apply to participate in the Medicare ACO programs [33].

While groups of providers with multiple TINs can apply collectively as a single ACO, the ACO must also have a single governing body that can contract with CMS. While CMS does not strictly define a minimum or maximum number of participating providers, applicant ACOs are expected to represent certain minimum thresholds of Medicare beneficiaries aligned with their providers. MSSP programs are expected to be accountable for 5,000 beneficiaries whereas Pioneer programs in non-rural areas must be accountable for 15,000 beneficiaries (see subsequent section for detail on how patients are "aligned" with Pioneer and MSSP programs) [34].

In 2011, CMS issued a request for applications to the Pioneer ACO program [35] and by the end of the year, CMS selected 32 organizations nationally to participate in the 3-year initiative, with an option at CMS' discretion to continue for two additional performance years if the program met its performance objectives [36]. In early 2014, CMS issued a request for information seeking feedback on a future Pioneer ACO solicitation and how the current cohort of Pioneer ACOs may evolve over time [37].

Under the MSSP program – a permanent program rather than a demonstration like the Pioneer – CMS has selected four cohorts of participants, two in 2011, one in 2012, and two in 2013, as well as recently closing a solicitation for 2014 applications [37]. MSSP agreements, like the Pioneer, cover three performance year periods [38]. To date, there are over 350 such ACOs, including some advanced payment ACOs, which is a variation of the MSSP program that includes some start up payments for ACO formation that are recouped out of shared savings, if achieved [38].

Patient Alignment and Engagement

Unlike a managed care or health plan model, beneficiaries do not enroll in an ACO. Rather, much like the PGP demonstration and the ACO concept as outlined by Dr. Fisher, defined populations of beneficiaries are aligned with particular ACOs. CMS has developed a methodology for analyzing individuals' historical utilization of particular Medicare providers and then determining primary healthcare providers to whom these individuals appear to be linked [39]. The intention of this imputed connection versus an enrollment model, is that it enables CMS to designate a locus of care responsible for coordinating a beneficiary's services, without in any way modifying the individual's network of providers. Aside from improved care coordination, beneficiaries assigned to an ACO should not observe changes to their benefit package or network of providers.

To align beneficiaries, CMS examines 3 years of historical service utilization data among Medicare FFS beneficiaries and then determines ACO applicant providers from whom beneficiaries have received the preponderance of their primary care (as determined through a list of "qualifying" Evaluation and Management codes). While the methodology focuses on isolating relationships between beneficiaries and primary care providers, CMS does incorporate beneficiary utilization of certain types of specialists such as nephrologists, oncologists, rheumatologists, endocrinologists, pulmonologists, neurologists, neuropsychiatrists, and cardiologists [39].

A key difference between the MSSP and Pioneer programs is that in the Pioneer program, ACOs can choose to have beneficiaries aligned prospectively. At the start of a performance year, Pioneer ACOs choosing this option will know the universe of beneficiaries for whom they will be fiscally and clinically responsible. A prospective alignment model enables Pioneer ACOs to target high cost, high need beneficiaries at the beginning of the performance year and manage their care throughout the entire period [40, 41].

By contrast, CMS uses retrospective alignment in the MSSP program, which is the approach that was also used in the PGP demonstration; Pioneer ACOs can also elect to have a retrospective alignment methodology, though it is not publicly known if any Pioneer ACOs have selected this option. Under the retrospective approach, CMS presents participating ACOs with a preliminary list of attributed individuals and then updates this list quarterly based upon actual service utilization until finalizing the alignment at the end of the performance year [41]. Retrospective alignment necessitates a broader population health strategy because ACOs do not know whom they will be financially responsible for in advance.

Financial Model

Both the MSSP and the Pioneer program are shared savings programs. If ACOs manage beneficiary healthcare costs beneath an expenditure benchmark, while meeting defined quality expectations, they can share in or access a portion of the dollars under the benchmark threshold. Regulation drafters sought to devise a shared savings methodology that would safeguard against inappropriate activities to bring down costs, like setting up barriers to access or reducing the quality of services, and protect against ACOs unfairly benefitting from overall trends in the market (e.g. a general national decline in Emergency Room utilization).

For the Pioneer and MSSP programs, CMS uses 3 years of average Medicare Part A and B expenditures for ACO-aligned beneficiaries to develop a financial benchmark [41]. In the MSSP program, the benchmark continues for the duration of the participation agreement with CMS (3 years) and similarly in the Pioneer program, the benchmark remains in place for 3 years and is recalculated in the fourth year of the demonstration. At a very high level, both programs take steps to adjust benchmarks for differential risk profiles of attributed beneficiaries, acknowledging that different age, sex, and disability sub-groups may incur very different expenditures [41]. Additionally, like the PGP demonstration, both programs have minimum savings rates (MSRs) that ACOs must surpass before accessing any savings or experiencing any losses; these MSRs are meant to protect against minor variations in expenditures year over year [41]. Underneath these general commonalties, there are a few key differences between the MSSP and Pioneer benchmark methodologies [41, 42]:

- **Risk Levels:** The Pioneer program involves greater levels of financial risk and savings opportunity in the initial years of implementation than the MSSP program and is therefore meant for organizations with prior experience executing ACO-like arrangements.
- **Population-Based Payments:** In the third year of the Pioneer demonstration (2014), certain ACOs were eligible to transition to a population-based payment, which involves receiving a portion of the FFS benchmark in advance on a monthly basis, similar to capitated payments. MSSP ACOs cannot access this payment option.
- **Performance-based payment contracts:** Pioneer ACOs are required to receive at least 50 % of their overall revenues through outcomes based payment arrangements such as shared savings deals; this requirement is premised upon the idea that if Pioneer ACOs substantially move their business model to such arrangements, it will better promote the triple aim. MSSPs do not have to meet this requirement, presumably because the model is focused on delivery systems with less risk experience.

Physician Payment

In the MSSP program and during the first 2 years of the Pioneer demonstration, physicians are paid as they usually are within the Medicare FFS program. However, as noted above, Pioneers that achieve certain levels of shared savings may receive population-based payments or pre-payments in the third year of the demonstration. With this flexibility, ACOs could theoretically choose to pay physicians differentially, though CMS has not indicated which if any ACOs had taken that step (physicians must also agree to participate in this payment structure). In the request for information released in early 2014, CMS solicited feedback from the field about evolving to ACO models with even greater levels of financial risk that would further enable ACOs to develop creative physician payment mechanisms [37].

Notably, the MSSP and Pioneer programs waive certain federal laws for the purposes of meeting the triple aim. Among other areas, ACOs are permitted to gainshare with participating providers [43]. Gainsharing, broadly speaking, is defined as delivery systems distributing savings accrued from cost reductions to healthcare providers who have helped generate those reductions. Typically, the Department of Health and Human Services has been wary of allowing such payments because such financial incentives could inappropriately induce physicians to limit patient care in order to cut down on costs [44]. In the context of the ACO program, however, such payments are expected to incentivize maximal coordination of patient care across settings, while quality performance standards safeguard against inappropriate reductions in care.

Quality Monitoring

In order to ensure that ACOs achieve cost reductions in a manner consistent with good clinical practice, CMS requires ACOs to meet several quality metrics, similar to the approach in the PGP demonstration. The 33 metrics in the MSSP and Pioneer program encompass a range of nationally accepted process and outcome metrics across the following four categories [45]:

- Patient/caregiver experience
- Care coordination/patient safety
- Preventive health
- At-risk population:
  - Diabetes
  - Hypertension
  - Ischemic Vascular Disease
  - Heart Failure
  - Coronary Artery Disease

For the most part, CMS selected measures from among those already used today in other CMS programs such as the Electronic Health Record (EHR) Incentive or the Physician Quality Reporting System programs. Even so, the ACO programs have offered an opportunity to advance the field of knowledge about these measures, in that a number have never previously been applied to a FFS population or have never been deployed nationally before. CMS is using findings from these programs to inform reasonable thresholds for quality performance [45].

Because of the experimental nature of several of the measures, shared savings are not immediately tied to actual quality performance by the ACOs. In the first year of the Pioneer demonstration and the first year of any MSSP initiation, ACOs are required to report on all quality metrics. In the second year, 25 of the 33 measures are "pay for performance," or impact the amount of savings retained, and finally in the third year, 32 of the 33 measures are pay for performance [45]. Performance is based upon patient survey data, claims and administrative data from CMS, and then data the ACOs must directly collect and report upon [46].

Care Coordination

Part of the rationale – if the not the most significant reason – for initiating ACO models at the federal level was a recognition that Medicare FFS beneficiaries are often subject to fragmented care. The Medicare Payment Advisory Commission has found that Medicare FFS beneficiaries frequently receive duplicative medical tests, receive inconsistent medical information or even different diagnoses from providers, and seek care from "higher-intensity" settings, like the emergency departments, than is warranted by their condition [47].

The ACO programs seek to address this fragmentation by stimulating groups of providers to better coordinate care for groups of FFS beneficiaries across healthcare settings. The federal programs promote better coordination through enabling gain-sharing amongst diverse providers, setting quality reporting and performance standards that embed cross-system collaboration, and requiring the establishment of governance structures that include representatives across a given delivery system or provider organization.

However, beyond those parameters, the ACO programs essentially defer to the participating providers to determine how to best coordinate care for beneficiaries – the models certainly do not call for particular clinical pathways or care management structures. With that latitude, ACOs have pursued a multiplicity of approaches to improve care coordination and reduce fragmentation. The following chapter provides a detailed case study of care management activities at Montefiore Medical Center, a Bronx, New York-based academic medical center that is implementing a Pioneer ACO model.

Other ACO Models

ACOs are not limited to the Medicare FFS program. ACOs have also proliferated nationally within Medicaid programs and amongst commercial payers. By some estimations, there are over 600 public and private payer ACOs nationally [48]. A number of state including Utah, Colorado, Oregon, and Minnesota have advanced models through their Medicaid programs designated to delegate financial and clinical risk to provider groups [49]. Managed care plans in some case have even advanced ACO like models, developing shared savings arrangements with contracted provider networks. As one example, Blue Cross Blue Shield of Massachusetts (BCBS) cultivated an alternative quality contracting (AQC) model through which it would provide a global budget to sub-contracted providers to manage all costs of their patients, while meeting quality targets. BCBS of Massachusetts worked closely with CMS in the development of the ACO programs, building upon lessons learned from the AQC model [50].

Conclusion

ACOs are not unicorns, but time will tell if they are in fact thoroughbreds – reliable cost-cutting, quality-enhancing programs, worthy of significant national expansion. Early information on the Medicare ACO programs is promising. Results from the first year of the Pioneer program showed that 13 of the 32 participating ACOs yielded $87.6 million in gross savings in 2012, translating into $33 million for the Medicare Trust Fund and shared savings amongst the Pioneers of $76 million (disclosure: Montefiore was the top financial performer amongst the Pioneer ACOs in the first demonstration year). Shared losses were more modest, totaling $4 million [51].

A subsequent independent analysis requisitioned by CMS that used a comparison group analysis instead of the benchmark methodology employed in the MSSP and Pioneer programs, also verified substantial savings associated with the two programs [52]. Little, however, is known about the infrastructure costs individual ACOs have incurred by instituting these programs or the structural features that increase the likelihood of clinical or financial success. More research and time is needed to fully appreciate the impacts of ACOs, both inside and outside the Medicare program. Notwithstanding that research gap – and the meandering path to our present day ACO models– what is evident is that the volume-driven FFS reimbursement framework once so foundational in the nation's healthcare system is slowly becoming a relic of days past.

References

1. Oberlander J. Political life of medicare. Chicago: University of Chicago Press; 2003.
2. National Bipartisan Commission on the Future of Medicare. The Medicare history page. Available at: http://rs9.loc.gov/medicare/history.htm. Accessed 9 Feb 2014.
3. Olakanmi O. The AMA and Medicare and Medicaid, 1965. American Hospital Association. Available at: http://www.ama-assn.org/resources/doc/ethics/medicare.pdf. Accessed 9 Feb 2014.
4. Burner ST, Davis MH. Three decades of Medicare: what the numbers tell us. Health Aff. 1995;14(4):231–43. Available at: http://content.healthaffairs.org/content/14/4/231.full.pdf. Accessed 9 Feb 2014.
5. Tufts Managed Care Institute. A brief history of managed care. Available at: http://www.thci.org/downloads/briefhist.pdf. Accessed 9 Feb 2014.
6. Jones and Bartlett Publishers. The origins of managed health care. Available at: http://www.google.com/url?sa=t&rct=j&q=&esrc=s&source=web&cd=1&cad=rja&ved=0CCYQFjAA&url=http%3A%2F%2Fwww.jblearning.com%2Fsamples%2F0763759112%2F59117_CH01_Pass2.pdf&ei=ZAn4UpWLIMPy0wGPsYCQDw&usg=AFQjCNFurY3vglSWoQxyAGMb3 0t1JjTGIw&bvm=bv.60983673,d.dmQ. Accessed 8 Feb 2014.
7. McGuire T, Newhouse J, Sinaiko A. An economic history of Medicare Part C. Milbank Q. 2011;89(2):289–32. Available at: http://www.ncbi.nlm.nih.gov/pmc/articles/PMC3117270/. Accessed 9 Feb 2014.
8. Thomas M, Uyehara E. Health maintenance organizations and the HMO Act of 1973. The Rand Corporation; 1975. Available at: http://www.rand.org/content/dam/rand/pubs/papers/2009/P5554.pdf. Accessed 9 Feb 2014.

9. Manning WG, Leibowitz A, Goldberg GA, Rogers WH, Newhouse JP. A controlled trial of the effect of a prepaid group practice on use of services. New Eng J Med. 1984;10(23):1505–10. Available at: http://www.ncbi.nlm.nih.gov/pubmed/6717541. Accessed 9 Feb 2014.
10. Medicare Payment Advisory Commission. Report to the congress: recent changes in the Medicare program, Chap 1. 2000. Available at: http://www.medpac.gov/publications/congressional_reports/Mar00%20Ch1.pdf. Accessed 9 Feb 2014.
11. The Henry J. Kaiser Family Foundation. Medicare advantage fact sheet. Available at: http://kff.org/medicare/fact-sheet/medicare-advantage-fact-sheet/. Accessed 9 Feb 2014.
12. Moon M, Gage B, Evans A. An examination of key provisions in the balanced budget act of 1997. Available at: http://www.commonwealthfund.org/Publications/Fund-Reports/1997/Sep/An-Examination-of-Key-Medicare-Provisions-in-the-Balanced-Budget-Act-of-1997.aspx. Accessed 9 Feb 2014.
13. Nicolson P. The effect of the balanced budget act of 1997 on Medicare HMO enrollment. University of Pennsylvania Population Aging Research Center; 2000. Available at: http://parc.pop.upenn.edu/sites/parc.pop.upenn.edu/files/parc/PARCwps00-01.pdf. Accessed 7 Feb 2014.
14. Melnick G, Shen Y. Is managed care still an effective cost containment device? 2005. http://www.usc.edu/schools/price/research/healthresearch/images/pdf_reportspapers/Managed_care_backlash_10_2005.pdf. Accessed 9 Feb 2014.
15. Biles B, Nicholas LH, Cooper BS, Adrion E, Guterman S. The cost of privatization: extra payments to Medicare advantage plans. 2006. http://www.commonwealthfund.org/Publications/Issue-Briefs/2006/Nov/The-Cost-of-Privatizatio--xtra-Payments-to-Medicare-Advantage-Plan--pdated-and-Revised.aspx. Accessed 7 Feb 2014.
16. Berenson R, Burton R. Accountable care organizations in Medicare and the private sector: a statusupdate.2011.http://www.urban.org/uploadedpdf/412438-Accountable-Care-Organizations-in-Medicare-and-the-Private-Sector.pdf. Accessed 1 Feb 2014.
17. Wilensky G. Lessons from the Physician Group Practice demonstration – a sobering reflection. New Eng J Med. 2011;365:1659–61. Available at: http://www.nejm.org/doi/full/10.1056/NEJMp1110185. Accessed 9 Feb 2014.
18. Trisolini M, Aggarwal J, Leung M, Pope G, Kautterx J. The Medicare Physician Group Practice demonstration: lessons learned on improving quality and efficiency in healthcare. 2008. http://www.commonwealthfund.org/~/media/Files/Publications/Fund%20Report/2008/Feb/The%20Medicare%20Physician%20Group%20Practice%20Demonstration%20%20Lessons%20Learned%20on%20Improving%20Quality%20and%20Effici/1094_Trisolini_Medicare_phys_group_practice_demo_lessons_learned%20pdf.pdf. Accessed 1 Feb 2014.
19. Ginsburg P. Bitter medicine: prescription to fix SGR requires a commitment to major medicare reform. Health Affairs Blog; 2008. Available at: http://healthaffairs.org/blog/2008/02/12/bitter-medicine-prescription-to-fix-sgr-requires-a-commitment-to-major-medicare-reform/. Accessed 5 Feb 2014.
20. Medicare Payment Advisory Commission (MedPAC). Washington, DC; 8 Nov 2006. Available at: http://www.medpac.gov/transcripts/1108_1109_medpac.final.pdf. Accessed 9 Feb 2014.
21. Gold J. ACO is the hottest three-letter word in health care. Kaiser Health News; 23 Aug 2013. Available at: http://www.kaiserhealthnews.org/stories/2011/january/13/aco-accountable-care-organization-faq.aspx. Accessed 2 Feb 2014.
22. The Patient Protection and Affordable Care Act; Public Law 111–148; 111th Congress. 23 Mar 2010. Available at: http://www.gpo.gov/fdsys/pkg/PLAW-111publ148/pdf/PLAW-111publ148.pdf. Accessed 2 Feb 2014.
23. The IHI Triple Aim. The Institute for Healthcare Improvement Web Site. Available at: http://www.ihi.org/engage/initiatives/tripleaim/pages/default.aspx. Accessed 9 Feb 2014.
24. Berenson RA, Cafarella N. The Center for Medicare and Medicaid innovation: activity on many fronts. 2012. Available: http://www.rwjf.org/en/research-publications/find-rwjf-research/2012/02/the-center-for-medicare-and-medicaid-innovation.html. Accessed 9 Feb 2014.
25. Medicare Shared Savings Program: Accountable Care Organizations (CMS-1345-P). Regulations.gov website. Available at: http://www.regulations.gov/#!documentDetail;D=CMS-2010-0259-0425. Accessed 9 Feb 2014.

26. Laws and Regulations. USA.gov web site. Available at: http://www.usa.gov/Topics/Reference-Shelf/Laws.shtml. Accessed 9 Feb 2014.
27. Office of the Federal Register. A guide to the rule making process. Available at: https://www.federalregister.gov/uploads/2011/01/the_rulemaking_process.pdf. Accessed 9 Feb 2014.
28. Center for Medicare and Medicaid Services. Pioneer accountable care organization request for application. Available at: http://innovation.cms.gov/Files/x/Pioneer-ACO-Model-Request-For-Applications-document.pdf. Accessed 9 Feb 2014.
29. Centers for Medicare and Medicaid Services. New affordable care act program to improve care, control Medicare costs, off to a strong start. 10 Apr 2014. Available at: https://www.cms.gov/apps/media/press/release.asp?Counter=4333&intNumPerPage=10&checkDate=&checkKey=&srchType=1&numDays=3500&srchOpt=0&srchData=&keywordType=All&chkNewsType=1%2C+2%2C+3%2C+4%2C+5&intPage=&showAll=&pYear=&year=&desc=false&cboOrder=date. Accessed 7 Feb 2014.
30. Physician Group Practice Transition Demonstration. Centers for Medicare and Medicaid Services web site. Available at: http://innovation.cms.gov/initiatives/Physician-Group-Practice-Transition/. Accessed 9 Feb 2014.
31. Johnson A. The model of the future? Wall Str J. 28 Mar 2011. Available at: http://online.wsj.com/news/articles/SB10001424052748703300904576178213570447994. Accessed 9 Feb 2014.
32. Centers for Medicare and Medicaid Services. Additional guidance for Medicare Shared Savings Program Accountable Care Organization (ACO) applicants. Available at: http://www.cms.gov/Medicare/Medicare-Fee-for-Service-Payment/sharedsavingsprogram/Downloads/Memo_Additional_Guidance_on_ACO_Participants.pdf. Accessed 9 Feb 2014.
33. Zezza MA. The final rule for the Medicare Shared Savings Program. Commonwealth Fund. Available at: http://www.commonwealthfund.org//media/Files/Publications/Other/2011/ZezzasummaryfinalruleMedicaresharedsavingsv2%202.pdf%29. Accessed 9 Feb 2014.
34. Boyarsky V, Parke R. The Medicare Shared Savings Program and the pioneer accountable care organizations. 2012. Available at: http://publications.milliman.com/publications/healthreform/pdfs/medicare-shared-savings-program.pdf.. Accessed 2 Feb 2014.
35. Center for Medicare and Medicaid Services. Request for information: evolution of ACO initiatives at CMS. Available at: http://innovation.cms.gov/Files/x/Pioneer-RFI.pdf. Accessed 5 Feb 2014.
36. Centers for Medicare and Medicaid Services. Pioneer Accountable Care Organization (ACO) model program frequently asked questions. Available at: http://www.google.com/url?sa=t&rct=j&q=&esrc=s&source=web&cd=1&cad=rja&uact=8&ved=0CDMQFjAA&url=http%3A%2F%2Finnovation.cms.gov%2FFiles%2Fx%2FPioneer-ACO-Model-Frequently-Asked-Questions-doc.pdf&ei=PJpdU8zuPKLa2AW9jIEw&usg=AFQjCNGTzsnZ9K2Qo6Ze15w3-zdrf4xgRw&bvm=bv.65397613,d.b2I. Accessed 27 Apr 2014.
37. Centers for Medicare and Medicaid Services Web Site. Available at: http://www.cms.gov/Medicare/Medicare-Fee-for-Service-Payment/sharedsavingsprogram/News.html. Accessed 9 Feb 2014.
38. Centers for Medicare and Medicaid Services. Advance payment Accountable Care Organization (ACO) model fact sheet. 2013. Available at: http://innovation.cms.gov/Files/fact-sheet/Advanced-Payment-ACO-Model-Fact-Sheet.pdf. Accessed 5 Feb 2014.
39. Centers for Medicare and Medicaid Services. Pioneer ACO alignment and financial reconciliation methods. Available at: http://innovation.cms.gov/Files/x/Pioneer-ACO-Model-Benchmark-Methodology-document.pdf. Accessed 7 Feb 2014.
40. Klar R. The importance of the shared savings ACO model. Health Affairs Blog; 2011. Available at: http://healthaffairs.org/blog/2011/01/25/the-importance-of-the-shared-savings-aco-model/. Accessed 9 Feb 2014.
41. Pyenson B, Fitch K, Iwasaki K, Berrios M. The two Medicare ACO programs: Medicare shared savings and pioneer – risk and actuarial differences. 2011. Available at: http://us.milliman.com/insight/health/The-two-Medicare-ACO-programs-Medicare-Shared-Savings-and-Pioneer-risk-and-actuarial-differences/. Accessed 1 Feb 2014.

42. Centers for Medicare and Medicaid Services. Pioneer Accountable Care Organization model: general fact sheet. 2012. Available at: http://innovation.cms.gov/Files/fact-sheet/Pioneer-ACO-General-Fact-Sheet.pdf. Accessed 3 Feb 2014.
43. Taking Advantage of Medicare ACO Waivers. The Advisory Board Company website. Available at: http://www.advisory.com/daily-briefing/2013/07/12/law-review. Accessed 9 Feb 2014.
44. Gainsharing. American Health Lawyers website. Available at: http://www.healthlawyers.org/hlresources/Health%20Law%20Wiki/Gainsharing.aspx. Accessed 9 Feb 2014.
45. RTI International and Telligen. Accountable Care Organization 2013 program analysis: quality performance standards narrative measure specifications. Available at: https://www.cms.gov/Medicare/Medicare-Fee-for-Service-Payment/sharedsavingsprogram/Downloads/ACO-NarrativeMeasures-Specs.pdf. Accessed 3 Feb 2014.
46. Trisolini M. Talk presented at academy health meeting. San Diego; 2013. Available at: http://academyhealth.org/files/2013/tuesday/trisolini.pdf. Accessed 4 Feb 2014.
47. Medicare Payment Advisory Commission (MedPAC) public meeting. Washington, DC; 8 Nov 2006. Available at: http://www.medpac.gov/transcripts/1108_1109_medpac.final.pdf. Accessed 9 Feb 2014.
48. Muhlestein D. Accountable care growth in 2014: a look ahead. Health Affairs Blog; 29 Jan 2014. Available at: http://healthaffairs.org/blog/2014/01/29/accountable-care-growth-in-2014-a-look-ahead/. Accessed 3 Feb 2014.
49. Kaiser Commission on Medicaid and the Uninsured. Emerging Medicaid Accountable Care Organizations: the role of managed care. 2012. Available at: http://kaiserfamilyfoundation.files.wordpress.com/2013/01/8319.pdf. Accessed 9 Feb 2014.
50. Alternative Quality Contract. Blue cross blue shield of Massachusetts web site. Available at: http://www.bluecrossma.com/visitor/about-us/affordability-quality/aqc.html. Accessed 9 Feb 2014.
51. Centers for Medicare and Medicaid Services. Pioneer Accountable Care Organizations succeed in improving care, lowering costs. Available at: http://www.cms.gov/Newsroom/MediaReleaseDatabase/Press-Releases/2013-Press-Releases-Items/2013-07-16.html. Accessed 9 Feb 2014.
52. Centers for Medicare and Medicaid Services. Medicare's delivery system reform initiatives achieve significant savings and quality improvements – off to a strong start. Available at: http://www.cms.gov/Newsroom/MediaReleaseDatabase/Press-Releases/2014-Press-releases-items/2014-01-30.html. Accessed 9 Feb 2014.

Chapter 5
Our Failing System: A Reasoned Approach Toward Single Payer

Ed Weisbart

Other than Quentin Young MD [1], physicians in the United States are an unhappy lot.[1] There are many explanations, but the bottom line is it's hard to be happy working in a profoundly dysfunctional system.

The percentage of American physicians who reported spending more than 5 h per week on paperwork and administration has skyrocketed from 47 % in 2012 to 80 % in 2013. More than a quarter of us now report spending more than 16 h per week in this way.[2] Fully 52 % of our primary care physicians report that the time required by them or their staff for pharmacy authorization is a major problem, compared to 21 % in Canada, 17 % in France, and 9 % in the United Kingdom.[3] No one went to medical school to become expert at shuffling paper.

The American health care system also fails to perform well in far more critical manners. Our life expectancy ranked 51st in 2013.[4] Health care is certainly not the only driver of life expectancy variations, but it is the one most directly under the influence of physicians. Americans are more likely to die of causes amenable to health care than in any other modern nation [2].

Our system also fails to perform financially. In 2011 our per capita health care expenditure was $8,950, roughly double that of any other modern nation. Canadians, for example, spent $4,780. In Great Britain, health care cost $3,280 per person.[5]

---

[1] Commonwealth Fund Survey of Primary Care Physicians. November 2012.
[2] Medscape – Physician Compensation Report.
[3] Commonwealth Fund Survey of Primary Care Physicians. November 2012.
[4] CIA World Fact Book, accessed Dec. 3 2013.
[5] OECD (2013).

E. Weisbart, M.D. (✉)
Internal Medicine, Barnes Jewish Medical Center,
618 N. New Ballas Road #305, Creve Coeur, MO 63141, USA
e-mail: edweisbart@gmail.com

Combine these two failures, and "American exceptionalism" takes on a dark meaning. The same data revealed that the Japanese spent $2,940 per capita, one third of what we spent, and yet their life expectancy was 11 years longer than ours.

According to an analysis of OECD data by Gerald Friedman, professor of economics at the University of Massachusetts-Amherst, up to 40 % of the variation in life expectancy among modern nations can be explained by how much each nation spends on health care. The United States is an exception in this; for our level of spending, we should be living 4 years longer than we do today. Or, we should be spending $6,700 less per person for our current life expectancy.[6] Either way, we're not getting results commensurate with the costs demanded by our system today.

Why are our costs so high? Is it the aging baby boom taking its toll? Is it our tobacco culture? Our obesity epidemic?

We happen to be among the younger of modern nations, and we smoke less than most others. Barely 13 % of us are over age 64. Nearly 15 % of Canadians, 16 % of British, and over 23 % of Japanese are aged.[7] While we have high rates of smoking in some states (my own state of Missouri boasts the lowest cigarette taxes in the nation and a smoking rate of 25 % among adults), as a nation less than 15 % of us smoke. 15.7 % of Canadians, 19.6 % of British, and 20.1 % of Japanese adults smoke.[8]

We lead the world in obesity, with over one third of us having a BMI above 30. We have already seen the direct consequences of growing rates of diabetes and hypertension, but we are just beginning to see the more expensive consequences of renal failure and cardiovascular diseases. Left unchecked, our leading position in obesity will clearly exacerbate the strain on our health care system, but does not explain our current situation.

Thirty seven percent of Americans report having cost-related problems accessing care; either they did not see a physician when sick, did not get some of the care that physician recommended, or they did not fill or skipped a medication because of cost. All other modern OECD nations report these problems at roughly one third (4–22 %) our current rate. Uninsured Americans fare the worst in the modern world, with 63 % reporting cost-related access problems. Those in the United States with health insurance do better, with only 27 % reporting these problems, but even that better number is still more than six times as high as Great Britain's 4 % rate [3].

Consumed by rising malpractice rates, collapsing reimbursements and increasingly bureaucratic demands on their time, physicians in the United States often fail to recognize their leadership opportunity to drive our national debate towards these real issues of health care. Physicians could recapture the moral high ground and advocate for equitable access to patient-centric care. A career in medicine makes

---

[6] Friedman, G. Presentations at PNHP-MO, March 2014.
[7] Ibid.
[8] Ibid.

physicians uniquely able to see how tragically easy it would be to better treat hypertension and prevent the high-cost strokes, heart attacks, and renal failure.

> One of my well-established hypertensives recently came in for an office visit with a blood pressure of 190/124. When I asked her what happened, she told me that she had three grandchildren living with her but could no longer afford both her rent and her medications. She had been homeless previously, felt she herself could bear that again, but refused to let her grandchildren experience that. She became tearful and asked me, "So, Dr. Weisbart, how long can I live without taking my blood pressure medicines?"

I never want to hear a question like that again.

> A colleague in Kentucky recently saw a 64 year-old woman with two obvious TIAs and an ipsilateral neck bruit. He recommended a full evaluation and possible endarterectomy, but she declined. She had no insurance and chose instead to "pray and wait" until turning 65 and getting Medicare.

Although we physicians hear these stories every day, our legislators seldom have direct access to them. Society grants physicians the privilege to hear these stories; it is therefore incumbent upon us to help our legislators understand how policy decisions that undermine universal access place American citizens (our grandmothers, friends, and neighbors) into untenable dilemmas. The voice of physicians is uniquely able to impact the dialogue.

Follow the Money

Professor Paul Batalden MD at Dartmouth famously once quipped, "Every system is perfectly designed to get the results it gets." Ours gets us excellence in technology but little drive towards public health.

We have chosen to put the health insurance industry at the center of American health care, yet the economics of the health insurance industry do not line up with advancing population health. Most insurers anticipate a 20–25 % turnover in annual membership as employers change insurers and patients change jobs. That means that they require a 2–4 year return on their investments in improving health, or they will be helping their competition. Most leaders in the industry are highly ethical and compassionate, but their fiduciary obligations would be violated by investing in health outcomes that don't deliver a return in that time frame.

We lead the world in virtually every metric of technology: CT scans and MRI exams, to name just two [4]. We have the best 5-year survival of virtually every type of cancer [5]. We have the world's highest rates of coronary bypass graft surgeries.[9]

Our business model drives us towards technology. An entrepreneurial physician can invest in a new imaging service, mechanical device, or specialty hospital and generate his or her own market demand. The Dartmouth Atlas Project has documented glaring variations in how medical resources are distributed and used in the

---

[9] OECD health data 2013.

United States. Much of this is more related to the availability of a service rather than the medical needs of a community. Most of the <variations in> spending was due to differences in use of the hospital… and to discretionary specialist visits and tests. Higher spending on these services does not appear to offer overall benefits [6].

In some ways, this is a source of tremendous pride for our nation. Our unequivocally strong results at treating diseases that require advanced technology are the envy of the world. Wealthy foreign nationals from countries with less robust health care technology are famous for visiting our tertiary care centers [7].

That same business model, unfortunately, does not align as strongly with the kinds of aggressive public health programs that are needed to improve the lives and life expectancies of our population. Our diabetics get more lower extremity amputations than those in almost any other nation.[10] We claim a "culture of life", yet our infant and maternal mortality rates rank worse than most other nations [4].

These are not problems that can be solved by building another imaging suite or opening another specialty hospital. They require the tireless hard work of primary care, prevention, education, lifestyle modification, and fundamental public health. They require access to health care, another vital area where the United States ranks worst among modern nations.[11]

Our costs are out of control for two big reasons – pricing and bureaucracy. A brilliant expose of how health care is priced in the United States consumed nearly the entire March 4 2013 issue of Time Magazine in an article by Steven Brill, "Bitter Pill: Why Medical Bills Are Killing Us [8]."

The pharmaceutical industry provides us with a microcosm of our system.

When Congress passed Medicare Part D, it included specific language barring the federal government from negotiating the prices of drugs. All one needs to know about the corrupting influence of money on politics is encased in that one sentence.

The retail price index for a basket of 2010 in-patent pharmaceuticals that cost $100 in the United States would cost $61 in France, $50 in Canada, and only $46 in the United Kingdom [9] . Per capita pharmaceutical spending the United States in 2011 was $995, more than double the average of other OECD nations. Canadian spending was $751. New Zealand spent under $300.[12]

One recent example illustrates many of the issues behind this.

In late 2013, the FDA approved Brisdelle, the first non-hormonal therapy for hot flashes associated with menopause. Hot flashes can be nearly disabling; a meaningfully improved treatment strategy would be welcome relief for millions. The new drug, Brisdelle, is a 7.5 mg formulation of paroxetine. Paroxetine is more familiar for its original branding as the antidepressant Paxil. With Paxil's patent long since expired, generic paroxetine is widely available at many community pharmacies for $4 per month.

---

[10] OECD Health Data 2013 (2009 or most recent available) per The Commonwealth Fund.
[11] Nolte E, op cit.
[12] Commonwealth Fund. Accessed Nov 28 2013.

The dose, however, is the critical factor. When used as an antidepressant, paroxetine was manufactured in dosages ranging from 10 to 40 mg, so those are the only dosage forms available for $4 per month.

Brisdelle is on the market at a slightly lower dosage, 7.5 mg. As that particular dosage of paroxetine was never approved for depression, there is no 7.5 mg strength of paroxetine on the market. It is difficult to believe there would be a clinically meaningful difference between 7.5 and 10 mg dosages in the safety or efficacy of treating menopausal hot flashes.

There is, however, quite a cost difference. Thirty tablets of 10 mg generic paroxetine are widely available for $4 per month; the same quantity of Brisdelle is priced at $150 for 30 tablets.[13]

In most circumstances today, pharmacists routinely offer patients a generic substitute if a physician writes for a brand name drug and does not indicate that such substitution is inappropriate. That substitution requires the pharmacist to have a generic that is FDA approved as chemically identical to the original prescription. As there is no direct generic equivalent to the 7.5 mg dosage form, a generic "substitution" would require the pharmacist or patient to call the prescriber and get an entirely new prescription. The time that work requires is onerous enough to frequently inhibit the effort.

Our bureaucracy is similarly unbridled. Between 1970 and 2010, we have seen a marginal growth in the number of physicians in the United States. In contrast, the number of administrators has increased by over 3,000 %. Health care marketing, contract negotiations and maintenance, information technology, etc. all drive medical overhead and administration, now considered to consume 31 % of our health care dollar. That means that a $1,300 monthly health insurance premium includes $400 for things that are unrelated to actual health care [10].

The diversion of these funds into the insurance industry also indirectly damages our nation's health. Families plagued by the rising cost of insurance are less able to send children to college. According to the County Health Calculator created by Steven Woolf MD, we would save 92,850 lives per year if 5 % more people had some college education and 4 % more had incomes higher than twice the federal poverty level. We would also prevent 915,000 cases of diabetes and eliminate $6.1 billion in diabetes costs every year [11]. Our uncontrolled system is not just making us poor, it's making us sick.

The core issue plaguing our health care system is the lack of alignment between the economic model we have chosen and the public health demands of our large and diverse nation. Unlike any other nation, we have chosen a market-based model of health care, wherein we juggle roughly 1,500 different insurance companies, government agencies, and others. This creates enormous redundancies and gaps, bureaucracies and Band-Aid solutions, a drive towards expensive yet insufficient insurance products, and extraordinary cost without extraordinary results. And it leaves tens of millions of us without any health insurance at all. Our healthcare system also poses barriers to communication and coordination of care.

---

[13] Brisdelle pricing from GoodRx.com, accessed Dec. 8, 2013.

The Affordable Care Act

These problems are partially mitigated by the Affordable Care Act. Vital new regulations of the insurance industry – guaranteed issue, ending rescissions and lifetime/annual maximums, etc. – are at long last accomplishing much of the Patient Bill of Rights [12]. Even the most aggressive opponents of the ACA favor retaining these features (Table 5.1).

However, the ACA will not do as well at addressing the financial challenges burdening most Americans. Sixty-two percent of bankruptcies in the United States are driven by medical expenses that make us more vulnerable to other economic insults, such as the 2008 recession and real estate collapse. Seventy-eight percent of medical bankruptcies occur among people who were insured at the onset of their bankrupting illness [13].

Many hope that the insurance reforms in the ACA will provide meaningful protection from medical bankruptcy, but the early evidence does not support that hope.

In 2008, Massachusetts implemented a state-wide health insurance reform even more generous than the ACA. In 2007, the year prior to implementation, Massachusetts saw 7,504 bankruptcies from medical expenses. In 2009 the number rose to 10,093 [14]. Much changed in the national economy during 2008, but at a minimum this evidence gives pause to the hope that the Affordable Care Act will end medical bankruptcies.

The value of the ACA's health insurance marketplaces is still emerging. Most users are expected to select a "silver" plan with an actuarial value of 70 %, leaving the individual responsible for 30 % of the cost of health care. The ACA may reduce the number of Americans without any insurance, but it is also normalizing under-insurance.

The expenses of starting and operating the ACA's health insurance marketplaces have already started to arrive and are anticipated to add roughly 3 % to our administrative burden. Vermont is anticipating 100,000 citizens to use their exchange, including 72,000 who had insurance before the ACA, at an initial cost of $170,000,000 or $6,071 per newly insured person. These numbers are exclusive of

Table 5.1 ACA's patient bill of rights

Ensuring coverage for consumers with pre-existing conditions
Ensuring the right to choose your doctor
Ensuring fair treatment when you need emergency care
Making sure your policy can't be canceled unfairly
Ending annual and lifetime limits
Enhancing access to preventive services
Ensuring your right to appeal health plan decisions
Ensuring health coverage for young adults
Protections under "Grandfathered Plans"

the additional $92,000,000 anticipated in 2015–2018 and $218,000,000 of additional costs over 5 years for integrated eligibility system, staffing, operations, etc.[14]

Other aspects of the ACA – information system adoption, payment model experiments, and delivery model innovations – are being widely adopted far in advance of a compelling business case. It remains speculative whether we can achieve improved population health and quality of care and limiting cost while retaining a private insurance model of health care finance.

In short, we receive modest benefits for an extraordinarily high cost system.

Lessons from Around the World

Every nation organizes their health care in a unique manner, but there are a handful of common principles. These are best summarized by the Canada Health Act's five main principles: Public administration, comprehensiveness, universality, portability, and accessibility [15].

- All modern nations other than the United States publicly administer their health insurance, much like Medicare is administered in the USA. They are typically accountable on a regional basis and are subject to regular public audits. Some nations, such as Germany, also involve highly regulated non-profit insurers.
- Rather than relying heavily on premiums, copays and deductibles, they are typically financed through their tax structure.
- All medically necessary health care services are comprehensively covered. This includes the primary and specialty physicians, mental health care, diagnostics, pharmaceuticals, ambulatory care, acute/emergent care, hospitalization, rehabilitation, and more.
- Every modern nation other than ours has found it feasible to provide these services to all citizens, often including non-citizen residents.
- Moving within the country – relocating to a different state or province – does not undermine the above guarantees.
- Lastly, single payer systems create the possibility of aligning facilities with the health care needs of the community. They are able to plan in such a way that all insured persons have reasonable access to health care facilities. As a corollary, all physicians and hospitals are provided reasonable compensation for their services.

Beyond these common characteristics, each nation has a unique blend of solutions. The broadest division among them is in how the delivery of care is organized. Many have chosen to preserve the private delivery of health care, where physicians and hospitals are free to organize themselves much as happens today in Canada. Those single payer systems are classified as "National Health Insurance" as the nationalization is focused on the insurance functions, not the delivery services.

---

[14] Independent Review of Health Benefits Exchange (HBE) and Integrated Eligibility (IE) Solutions, July 2013.

In addition to nationalizing the insurance functions, other countries have also nationalized their delivery model. These "National Health Service" forms of single payer typically see physicians directly employed by the national government. The prototype for this model is in Great Britain, where specialists are employed by the government. Most primary care physicians in Great Britain remain privately organized but carry national contracts [16]. The closest version of this in the United States would be the way care is organized within our Veterans Administration, where both primary and specialty care physicians are employed directly.

Medicare Today

Prior to 1965, less than 50 % of seniors had health insurance and were frequently thrown into poverty, disability, or premature death. They were not generally included in employer-sponsored plans, and the commercial insurance industry considered them "bad risks". The Social Security Administration identified the high cost of medical care as the greatest single cause of economic dependency in old age [17].

By 1965, with the continued aging of the country and escalation of both hospital costs and insurance premiums, two-thirds of the nation supported the passage of Medicare. "Public confidence in the social security system was an important contributing factor; many advocates made a point of stressing that Medicare would utilize the "tested" and "proven" mechanism of social security [18]."

Medicare continues to prove its popularity among Americans across a diverse range of people. A recent poll showed that 76 % of Americans, and 62 % of self-identified Tea Party members, agreed that "the benefits from government programs such as Social Security and Medicare are worth the costs."[15]

Part of the popularity of Medicare is due to its meeting many of the above criteria: Public administration, comprehensiveness, universality, portability, and accessibility. A private market has emerged to fill the gaps between those goals and what Medicare actually provides today.

Publicly administered, Medicare does not have to carry many of the costs inherent in the commercial insurance industry.

Private insurance companies typically offer hundreds or thousands of different benefit packages, combining variations in copayments, networks, formularies, approvals, and promotional materials. This market-driven structure requires an exhaustive and highly redundant commitment in human resources and capital investment. The business demands driving this effort are more clearly aligned with the insurers' fiduciary obligations than improving the health of the population. Medicare offers a single benefit design for all beneficiaries, enabling a far greater percentage of its resources to be devoted to paying for care. For example, managed

---

[15] CBS News/New York Times poll, April 14, 2010.

care companies reported overhead rates of 16.1–26.6 % in the first half of 2013,[16] whereas Medicare operates with a roughly 2 % overhead.

Privately administered health insurance policies have arcane exclusions and restrictions that are virtually impossible for patients to understand until they discover in their moment of need. And then it is too late to turn to the free market for a new product. They regularly categorize high-expense medical procedures as non-covered benefits under the dual dark umbrellas of "experimental" or "cosmetic".

Seventeen year-old Natalie Sarkisyan's death in 2007 made headlines when Cigna HealthCare denied the request from multiple physicians to perform a liver transplant to treat a complication from her recurrent leukemia. Cigna ultimately reversed the denial after a great deal of media attention, but she died a few hours later [19].

It is beyond our scope to analyze whether the denial or approval of her transplant was medically justified. The reversal under intense public attention, however, exposes the arbitrary nature of many insurance company benefit determinations. They justified their initial denial of payment based upon language in their benefits documentation; they classified the procedure as "experimental" and therefore not among the services Ms. Sarkisyan's family purchased when paying insurance premiums. The family ultimately sued Cigna but the case was thrown out of court due to previous Supreme Court rulings that shield employer-paid healthcare plans from damages over their coverage decisions [20].

The health insurance industry favors its chief executives with generous compensation packages. In 2012, Coventry' CEO Allen Wise received $12.0 million; Cigna's David Cordani received $12.9 million; United HC's Steve Hemsley received $13.9 million; Wellpoint's Angela Braly received $20.6 million; and Aetna's Mark Bertolini was graced with $113.3 million.[17] In contrast, the president of the United States of America has an annual salary of $400,000. Sylvia Mathews Burwell, US Secretary of Health and Human Services, earns less than half that amount ($199,700).

At least in health care, public administration is a bargain.

Despite its efficiencies, Medicare is an imperfect solution today, even for those who depend upon it. Most seniors have found that the current Medicare benefit design does not fully meet their needs. Several medically needed services – nutrition, dental, durable medical equipment, vision, hearing, and long-term care – are simply not included in the benefit design. They also learn that Medicare includes significant cost-sharing, with inpatient deductibles over $1,200, monthly premiums for Part B of over $100, and income-adjusted premiums for the optional drug benefit [21].

Seniors often purchase Medicare supplemental insurance from a private insurer to bridge some of the coverage gaps identified above. In addition, many purchase a wrap-around policy to cover their deductibles and co-insurance.

These common purchases identify the market's voice about the limitations of the current Medicare program and can be used to identify needed improvements.

---

[16] SEC Filings/Reports to Shareholders for Q1-Q2 of 2013. Calculated as 100 % – Medical Loss Ratio.

[17] Modern Healthcare. May 13 2013.

Medicare Tomorrow: A Solution Hiding in Plain Sight

The most obvious difference between the United States health care system and those in virtually every other modern nation has to do with the financial structure of funding and distribution. While there are countless variations, the rest of the modern world uses a "single-payer" system in which "a single public or quasi-public agency handles all health care financing. Delivery of care may remain in public or private hands, depending on the particular system [22]."

Other than the Affordable Care Act, the most popular piece of health care legislation in the recent history of the United States Congress is HR676, "The Expanded and Improved Medicare for All Act." First introduced by Representative John Conyers (D-MI) in 2003 with 25 co-sponsors, as of this writing the bill enjoys 58 co-sponsors. In short, this act would correct the shortcomings of the current Medicare program and provide it to all Americans, regardless of age. Several economic analyses show that this would be far less expensive than our current fragmented multi-payer model, while providing universal access to comprehensive care.

Although HR676 is unlikely to ever pass unchanged into law, it serves as a "North Star", identifying broad strategic solutions to many of the structural problems inherent in today's environment.

Key Provisions of HR676

- Patients would have freedom of choice of clinicians and hospitals. No longer would patients need to consult their insurer's directory, as virtually all providers would be "in network". Rather than today's model that drives physicians and hospitals to "optimize their payer mix" by shunning low-reimbursement insurers, all patients would represent equal economic opportunities for physicians and hospitals.
- Comprehensive benefits, including primary care, subspecialty care, prevention, dietary and nutritional therapies, inpatient care, outpatient care, emergency care, prescription drugs, durable medical equipment, long-term care, palliative care, mental health services (at parity with medical services), full non-cosmetic dental, substance abuse treatment, chiropractor, basic vision, hearing and hearing aids, and podiatry. Insurers are prohibited from selling health insurance coverage that duplicates the benefits provided under HR676.
- Institutions are required to be public or non-profit, with compensation to owners for reasonable financial losses incurred as a result of the conversion to non-profit status. Private physicians and clinics can continue to operate as private entities but are prohibited from being investor-owned.

- Having a single payer enables a rational approach to health care budgeting, key to long-term cost control.
    - Three discrete non-fungible annual budgets would be established:
        - Operating budget for optimal health care professional staffing. Clinicians could be reimbursed either through fee for service or salaried positions. Interest would be due providers not reimbursed within 30 days of claims submission;
        - Capital expenditures budget for construction or renovation of health facilities, and major equipment purchases;
        - Health professional education budget, including continued funding of physician training programs.
    - Co-mingling these budgets would be prohibited, thus preventing hospitals from funding market-driven expansions and equipment purchases by decreasing their nurse:patient formulas.
    - Global budgets would be set through annual negotiations between providers and regional directors.
- The prices of pharmaceuticals, medical supplies, and assistive equipment would be negotiated nationally on an annual basis. A single prescription drug formulary, open to petition by physicians and patients, would encourage best-practices. Physicians today often need familiarity with several dozen formularies, undermining their ability to deepen their knowledge of their most-needed medications.
- The program would be funded by a new Medicare for All Trust Fund, combining current federal health care funding with modest increases in personal income taxes for the top 5 % of earners, excise taxes on payroll and self-employment, unearned income, and stock and bond transactions.
- The single payer system would reduce expenses through vastly reduced paperwork, bulk procurement as mentioned above, and improved access to preventive health care.
- The program would be administered through coordinated regional and state governance.
- A National Board of Universal Quality and Access would represent health care professionals, institutional providers of care, representatives of health care advocacy groups, labor unions, and citizen patient advocates, all without conflicts of interest. Among other things, twice a year they would address access to care, quality improvement, efficiency of administration, adequacy of budget and funding, appropriateness of provider reimbursements, capital expenditures, and staffing levels and working conditions in health care delivery facilities.
- Clerical, administrative, and billing personnel whose jobs are eliminated due to reduced administration would have first priority at retraining and job placement in the new system, and be eligible to receive 2 years of employment transition benefits with salary guarantee up to $100,000 per year, and then be eligible to begin unemployment benefits if not employed.

The New Savings from a Single Payer Model Would Outweigh the New Expenses

New annual costs would total $326 billion ($74 billion from normalizing provider payments for Medicaid patients, $110 billion for covering the uninsured, and $142 billion from increased utilization, particularly home health and dental.) New annual savings would total $569 billion ($23 billion in government administration, $153 billion in health insurance administration, $178 billion from increased ability to negotiate the prices of drugs and devices, and $215 billion from administrative cost reductions for providers). The net savings from a single payer program are thus estimated at $243 billion, covering everyone with better benefits and spending less overall.[18]

By shifting from deductibles, co-insurance, and other financial barriers to care to a tax-based model, 95 % of Americans would spend less on health care under this model.[19]

Single Payer Would Level the Global Business Playing Field for Employers and Labor

Employers would be able to book reductions in costs and rely upon other reduced financial risks.

In addition to the direct cost of the actual health benefit (8–11 % of payroll costs) they would no longer provide, benefit administration by itself is complex, expensive (up to 3.2 % of current spending) (Friedman, personal communication) and not necessary under a single payer model. The ever-growing costs of providing health care to entitled retirees would disappear. There would be concomitant reductions in the cost of Workers Compensation, liability, and automobile insurance.

The future cost of business would become more predictable, insulated from the dramatic swings that can occur today. This is particularly important for smaller employers, where one illness, one premature baby, one cancer, one major automobile accident, can dramatically increase their expense that year. The risk of hiring a new employee with unrecognized medical needs would disappear. They would have fewer disincentives for hiring productive but older and less-healthy workers. Finally, there would be one less item on the labor negotiation table, making it simpler to focus on wages.

As much as half of the slowdown in wages increases since 1973 is due to higher health insurance premiums. Health insurance divides labor, pitting young and health workers against those older and less healthy.

---

[18] Friedman, G. Dollars and Sense. March/April 2012.
[19] Ibid.

The Roads to Single Payer

The Affordable Care Act has for the first time in our nation's history established a legislative commitment to providing all Americans with access to affordable health care. While the ACA itself does not fully achieve this lofty goal, the commitment itself is a milestone to be celebrated.

We could pursue something akin to single payer by expanding the ACA's regulation of the insurance industry. Maryland has embarked on this road with uniform hospital price structures. Expanding this model could achieve an "all-payer" program akin to Germany or Switzerland. Noted health care futurist Uwe Reinhardt has advocated for this model, stating:

> An all-payer system with multiple private insurers would be likely to be more broadly politically feasible than a government-run single-payer system, such as Canada's provincial, government-run single-payer insurance systems. A single-payer system, of course, would be another alternative that would eliminate price discrimination and any cost shifting. [23]

Given how fiercely the health insurance industry would oppose adoption of an all-payer system in the United States, our political efforts would be better spent towards the more comprehensive solutions inherent in true single-payer models.

The legislative process is seldom linear [24]. Rather than expect HR676 to pass in one single leap, the more likely pathways are through strategic incrementalism. In some ways, the United States has already embarked down this road, ensuring health care access for seniors, children, veterans, and other groups. We are also committed to providing coverage for perceived high-value medical conditions such as renal dialysis, amyotropic lateral sclerosis, and a wealth of other conditions often mandated by individual states. We could continue down this path, narrowing the age gap between SCHIP and Medicare programs, adding more high-value conditions and treatments, and identifying additional populations to protect.

Canada began their path to universal health care in a single province, Saskatchewan. After a very stormy beginning, the federal government offered support to any Canadian province that followed the Saskatchewan model and met a handful of characteristics. Within a few short years, it had become a profound success across their nation and is now treasured by most Canadians.

A parallel path is possible within the United States. The Affordable Care Act permits individual states to opt out of much of the structure within the ACA, as long as the alternative they propose covers more of their citizens and is better at controlling costs. The ACA allows HHS to grant these waivers beginning in 2017. The Vermont legislature has enacted the first steps towards this option, with the full support of their governor.

While a state-based reform is an incomplete solution and not truly a "single payer" model, it is as close an approximation as is supported by current federal legislation and will bring much broader access at tremendous savings. Many other states have been making initial steps down the same road. The first states to implement this will enjoy a stimulated economy, resources freed up for other vital functions such as education, and strong competitive advantages at attracting businesses from less progressive states.

A third strategy would be to add the "public option" into the ACA's insurance exchanges and then gradually migrate existing public programs. Eventually, the demand for private insurance would become increasingly rarefied and a single payer could emerge.

One additional scenario would be to improve Medicare in the manner described above, provide it to all children under age 18, and lower the age of eligibility for adults to 55 years. Over time, the gap between the age limits could be narrowed and eventually closed, achieving universal coverage.

While these incremental strategies may be more readily achievable, they each fail to deliver the fundamentally transformative power of a true single payer until they reach the last step along their pathways. Clearly, the most elegant strategy is to simply pass HR676 and provide universal access to comprehensive health care, prevent tens of thousands of needless deaths every year, and quickly improve the ability of American businesses to compete in the global marketplace.

Many physicians want and need to lead our country to single payer. Multiple surveys over the past 14 years have documented a growing majority of American physicians prefer a single payer model to our current system. The most recent data come from Maine [25], where an impressive 64.3 % of survey respondents said they would prefer a single-payer system, up from 52.3 % in 2008 when exactly the same language was used. Similar trends have been seen in Massachusetts [26], Minnesota [27], and nationwide [28].

Our profession must more fully act upon our responsibility to improve the health and well-being of our nation. "It took me until middle age to realize the importance of advocating for my patients *outside* of the exam room (Steve Keithahn, 2013, personal communication)."

At the End of the Day

Single payer does not represent a magical panacea that would cure all of the ills with our nation's health care system. It does, however, establish an alignment between health outcomes and economic performance. In doing so, it would be the first step in a series of innovations and reforms that would help the United States recover its role as a global leader. The sooner we start, the sooner we improve.

References

1. Young Q. Everybody in, nobody out. Copernicus Healthcare, Friday Harbor, WA. 2013.
2. Nolte E, McKee M. Variations in amenable mortality – trends in 16 high-income nations. Health Policy (published online 12 Sept 2011). http://www.commonwealthfund.org/publications/in-the-literature/2011/sep/variations-in-amenable-mortality.
3. Schoen C, et al. Access, affordability, and insurance complexity are often worse in the United States compared to ten other countries. Health Aff. 2013;32(12):2205–15.

4. http://www.oecd.org/els/health-systems/oecdhealthdata2013-frequentlyrequesteddata.htm. Accessed 17 Feb 2014.
5. http://www.cancer.org/acs/groups/content/@epidemiologysurveilance/documents/document/acspc-027766.pdf. Accessed 28 Nov 2013.
6. www.dartmouthatlas.org. Accessed 2 Feb 2014.
7. http://www.kttc.com/story/24452019/2014/01/15/saudi-arabian-airlines-jetliner-brings-visitors-for-10-day-rochester-visit. Accessed 17 Feb 2014.
8. Brill S. Bitter pill: why medical bills are killing us. Time Mag. 4 Mar 2013. Retrieved from: http://time.com/#198/bitter-pill-why-medical-bills-are-killing-us/
9. Kanavos P, et al. Higher US branded drug prices and spending compared to other countries may stem partly from quick uptake of new drugs. Health Aff. 2013;32(4):753–61.
10. Woolhandler S, et al. Costs of Health Administration in the U.S. and Canada. NEJM. 21 Sept 2003;349(8).
11. http://countyhealthcalculator.org/location/100000/. Accessed 16 Mar 2014.
12. The Affordable care Act: Patient's Bill of rights and other protections, Families USA brief. 2011. Retrieved from: http://familiesusa.org/sites/default/files/product_documents/Patients-Bill-of-Rights.pdf and contained in: http://www.cms.gov/CCIIO/Programs-and-Initiatives/Health-Insurance-Market-Reforms/Patients-Bill-of-Rights.html
13. Himmelstein D, et al. Medical bankruptcy in the United States, 2007: results of a national study. Am J Med. 2009.
14. Himmelstein DU, Thorne D, Woolhandler S. Medical bankruptcy in massachusetts: has health reform made a difference? Am J Med. 2011;124:224–228.
15. Canada Health Care. http://www.canadian-healthcare.org/page2.html. Accessed 17 Feb 2014.
16. http://www.commonwealthfund.org/~/media/Files/Publications/Fund%20Report/2013/Nov/1717_Thomson_intl_profiles_hlt_care_sys_2013_v2.pdf. Accessed 17 Feb 2014.
17. http://www.ssa.gov/history/corningchap4.html. Accessed 18 Feb 2014.
18. http://www.ssa.gov/history/corningchap4.html. Accessed 17 Feb 2014.
19. Chen PW. When insurers put profits between doctor and patient. The New York Times. 6 Jan 2011.
20. Girion L. Insurer's agreement to cover surgery comes too late. Los Angeles Times. 2009. www.articles.latimes.com. Accessed 8 Oct 2012.
21. http://www.medicare.gov/your-medicare-costs/costs-at-a-glance/costs-at-glance.html#collapse-4811. Accessed 18 Feb 2014.
22. Drasga R, Einhorn L. Why oncologists should support single-payer national health insurance. Am Soc Clin Oncol. 2013. Jop.ascopubs.org
23. Reinhardt U. The many different prices paid to providers and the flawed theory of cost shifting: is it time for a more rational all-payer system? Health Aff. 2011;30(11):2125–33.
24. Johnson H, Broder D. The system: the american way of politics at the breaking point. Back Bay Books, Little, Brown and Company. Boston, New York, London. 1997.
25. Maine Medical Association. Payment reform survey – MMA resolution questions. http://www.mainemed.com/sites/default/files/content/Payment%20Reform%20Survey%20-%20%28Crescendo%29.pdf. Accessed 18 Mar 2014.
26. Worcester Business Journal Online. http://www.wbjournal.com/article/20111107/PRINTEDITION/311079986. Accessed 18 Mar 2014.
27. Albers J, et al. Minnesota medicine. http://www.minnesotamedicine.com/PastIssues/PastIssues2007/February2007/ClinicalHealthCareFebruary2007/tabid/1709/Default.aspx. Accessed 18 Mar 2014.
28. Carroll A, Ackerman R. Support for national health insurance among U.S. physicians: 5 years later. Ann Intern Med. 2008;148(7):566–7.

Chapter 6
Geriatric and Primary Care Workforce Development

Michael R. Wasserman

There has been considerable concern as to whether the physician workforce will be adequate in the coming years [1]. Perhaps the more pertinent, and specific, question is related to what is needed from the healthcare workforce in the United States in the coming years as the population continues to age? Will there be an adequate supply of health care providers? Will they have the necessary skills? Will they be the appropriate type of providers and will they be properly trained to care for the growing number of older people? Numbers alone do not provide all of the answers. The demographics are well known, and they provide a striking contrast to historical health care workforce needs. In 1900, there were 3.1 million Americans age 65 and older. Today, that number is close to 40 million. By 2030, 20 % of all Americans will be over the age of 65. People age 85 and older are the fastest growing segment of the entire population, with expected growth from four million people today to 19 million by 2050. The rapid growth in older people in the United States begs the question about whether our health care workforce is prepared for this growth.

Prior to 1910, the development of our health care workforce historically had been one defined predominantly by reactions to market forces [2]. After the Flexner report in 1910, there was an increase in professionally dominated regulation but the geographic distribution of physicians followed market needs [2]. Since the implementation of the Medicare program in 1965, the development of a workforce to care for the older population has not responded based on market forces and we are now facing a significant shortage. We will explore some of the possible reasons for this workforce shortage and discuss potential solutions to this growing problem. Any discussion of the physician workforce necessary to care for our aging population must also begin and end with a discussion of the field of geriatric medicine. As geriatrics is a relatively new specialty, it also makes sense to first look at the

M.R. Wasserman, M.D. (✉)
Division of Geriatric Medicine, University of Colorado Denver,
22912 Erwin St., Woodland Hills, CA 91367, USA
e-mail: wassdoc@aol.com

historical development of other specialties in order to gain some insight in regards to the lack of development of geriatrics. Ironically, the specialty that makes sense both from a historical demographic perspective and practice perspective is pediatrics.

At the turn of the twentieth century, pediatrics was a relatively new specialty that existed primarily in academic institutions. Over time, pediatricians put up their shingles and the free market responded. Pediatrics entered the realm of board certification in the 1930s along with a number of other specialties. Today, many parents take their children to a pediatrician. Ironically, the first major growth in pediatrics probably occurred during the 1940s and 1950s, when todays "baby boomers" were born and there were many advances in medical science. By the tail end of this period, however, general pediatrics had lost its luster as the focus drifted away from the challenges of treating illness to a greater focus on wellness and prevention [3]. This coincided with a decline in income compared to other medical specialties. It is notable that despite these factors, the number of pediatricians in the United States has continued to increase over the past 20 years. Today there are well over 50,000 actively practicing pediatricians in the United States [4].

Pediatrics and other specialities seem to have historically responded to market needs. The specialty of geriatrics has definitely not taken the same path, despite a demographic imperative that has seen an unprecedented growth in the number of older people in the United States, fueled by the same baby boomer population that fueled the growth of pediatrics. Numerous studies have suggested that in the coming years there will be a need for well over 20,000 geriatricians [5]. Not only are the present number of geriatricians far below the present and expected need, but the number has actually been declining. There appears to be multiple reasons for this. The methods for the financing of physician training and determining physician reimbursement appear to be two of the major factors in the equation. We will first take a look at how the financing of physician training might have an impact on the development of geriatricians.

Prior to 1965, after graduating from medical school a physician would typically enter a 1 year internship. Often, this internship would consist of experiences in all of the major fields of medicine, such as internal medicine, pediatrics, surgery and obstetrics. After 1 year of internship, some physicians would put up a shingle as a general practitioner. Others would go on to complete residencies in the aforementioned fields. Interns would work very long hours and were generally compensated only with room and board [6]. The incentive to get out and work was fairly high. This all changed in 1965, when the Medicare program came into existence.

With the passing of the Medicare legislation, there were concerns as to whether a new health insurance program for older people would put a strain on the physician workforce (there are interesting similarities in regards to concerns about the Affordable Care Act). There were actually concerns as to whether there would be an adequate workforce to care for the growth in the older population in the coming years. The concept of public funding of graduate medical education grew out of this concern as congress saw the need to support medical education. It was legislated that this funding would come out of the Medicare Trust Fund. The theory was pretty straightforward. The growth of a new program ensuring health care for older adults would also require the growth of a physician workforce necessary to provide the health care for this population. Public funding of Graduate Medical Education (GME) was meant to assure the future growth in the physician workforce by making it easier for doctors to get through their training. Over the last 49 years, this support has continued to grow.

In 2012, the Medicare Trust Fund spent over $10 billion in the direct and indirect support of GME [7]. The result of this experiment in attempting to engineer the growth of the physician workforce is decidedly mixed. Over the past 49 years we have definitely seen the growth of the physician workforce overall, but the development of the very physicians (and other health care professionals) who are needed to provide health care to older individuals is clearly inadequate. We will explore some of the possible reasons for this. Some point to legislation in the Balanced Budget Act of 1997 that capped the number of residents that hospitals could have as the turning point for physician workforce issues. Cooper, in fact, stated "There has never been an action affecting medical education that has had as broad a consensus, yet it was this single action, now repudiated by many of its signatories, that fully accounts for the physician shortages that are now being encountered" [1]. While the number of geriatricians in the United States peaked around this time, the problem is far more complex than being linked solely to a cap on residents, as can be seen by the continuing disparity between physicians choosing to become specialists versus those choosing to devote their careers to primary care, which includes a career in geriatrics.

The methods by which the government determines both direct and indirect GME funding has numerous implications on both workforce needs and care delivery in the settings that this funding is provided, and subsequently to the community. Over the past 15 years there have been several studies documenting the complexity and lack of accountability with the present GME structure [8]. While there has clearly been a need for more primary care trainees, the GME funding structure itself has discouraged primary care programs in relation to more procedure oriented specialties. Hospitals tend to favor procedure oriented specialties as they tend to bring in more revenue. In response to this trend, the Council on Graduate Medical Education (COGME) has consistently called for increased GME funding as a means to achieve an increase in primary care trainees. One could see how this might just lead to throwing additional money into the same situation that we presently have. The question that begs to be asked is how additional funding will reverse the trend towards specialty and procedure driven care without a change to the existing structure and incentives under which the GME program operates.

One of the other major problems with the public funding of physician training is that the subsidization of GME through the use of Medicare funds has never truly focused on preparing the physician workforce to care for the older population that the Medicare program primarily serves. In the beginning, this certainly reflected the actual development of the field of geriatrics in the United States. While the term "geriatrics" was coined in 1909 by Ignatz L. Nascher, the American Geriatrics Society ("AGS") wasn't founded until 1942, and really didn't even begin to start growing until many years later [9]. The first geriatric fellowship program didn't open until 1966, just 1 year after the founding of the Medicare program. It wasn't until 1977 that the first Professorship in Geriatrics in the United States was established at Cornell University. The first Department of Geriatrics at a major teaching center, Mount Sinai Medical School, didn't open until 1982. With the slow development of geriatrics as a defined entity, there was very little ability to even consider developing expectations for geriatric competencies in medical education in concert with the funding of GME. Unfortunately, a robust academic presence of geriatrics has yet to develop in medical schools across the country. In fact, there are only six Geriatric Departments today in medical schools throughout the United States [9]. In 2009 there was finally some agreement on core geriatric competencies for medical school graduates [10]. How these competencies are incorporated into medical schools has yet to be determined [11].

Should geriatrics even be its own specialty? It is reasonable to ask whether the lack of development of geriatric medicine is related to a lack of a need for the specialty. When Dr. Nascher coined the term geriatrics, he described it as "an addition to our vocabulary, to cover the same field in old age that is covered by the term pediatrics in childhood, to emphasize the necessity of considering senility and its diseases apart from maturity and to assign it a separate place in medicine." Five years later he wrote the first American textbook on geriatric medicine, Geriatrics: The Diseases of Old Age and Their Treatment, Including Physiological Old Age, Home and Institutional Care, and Medico-Legal Relation [12]. The focus was primarily on the issues faced by aging individuals at the time.

Following the lead of Drs. Nascher and Marjorie Warren (in Great Britain), the early focus of geriatric medicine leaned more towards addressing socioeconomic issues such as debility, chronic care and institutionalization [13]. While the clinical approach to internal medicine has historically focused on diagnosis, treatment and cure, geriatric medicine has tended to focus on quality of life and function. The same principals laid out in the GeriMed Philosophy of Care [14] (noted in chapter 8) (Table 6.1) are an excellent description of the varying facets of geriatric medical care and are consistent with other descriptions of geriatrics in the literature [15].

Table 6.1 GeriMed philosophy of care	
	Focus on function
	Focus on managing chronic disease(s) and developing chronic care treatment models
	Identify and manage psychological and social aspects of care
	Respect patient's dignity and autonomy
	Respect cultural and spiritual beliefs
	Be sensitive to the patient's financial condition
	Promote wellness
	Listen and communicate effectively
	Patient centered approach to care, customer focused approach to service
	Realistically promote optimism and hope
	Team approach to care

Since the time of Dr. Nascher, there has been a recognition amongst geriatricians that older individuals may require a different approach to care than younger patients. There has also been an intuitive understanding amongst geriatricians that older patients may not only respond differently to illnesses than their younger counterparts, but that the treatment needs of older people might be different. While the last 50 years has seen a growth in research on the aging process, there has been a definite lag in the clinical research comparing the treatment needs of older people to the younger population. In fact, many clinical research trials have historically excluded patients over the age of 75. Some have tried to separate out specific "geriatric syndromes" and develop research and policy approaches based on this concept [16]. Others have pointed out the differences in approaches to caring for a broad variety of clinical conditions as people age [17]. The term "gerogeriatrics" has recently been coined to recognize that in the oldest old clinicians approach diseases such as diabetes and hypertension in a fashion that is different than their approach to younger individuals [18]. The fact of the matter is that aging is a continuum and these differences certainly occur at some point along this continuum. Recognizing these changes and adjusting our diagnostic and treatment approaches to account for them is the realm of the geriatrician and other geriatric health care professionals.

Focusing on a set of specific clinical syndromes or addressing the socioeconomic challenges of aging is too limiting of an approach to defining geriatrics. In the last decade there have been a number of studies that have lent credence to the fact that older people might need to be treated differently than their younger counterparts. One of the first such clinical trials, the AFFIRM study, demonstrated that the treatment of atrial fibrillation in the elderly was different than in younger individuals. In older patients, the use of cardioversion and antiarrhythmic medications in trying to treat and prevent atrial fibrillation has been shown to be associated with worse outcomes than in younger patients [19].

Recently, it has become clear that aggressive treatment of elderly men for prostate cancer may be more harmful than conservative treatment [20]. In fact, in my personal experience over the past 25 years, I have only seen two men over the age of 80 die from prostate cancer. It is likely that both of these men had the disease prior to turning 70. While there are certainly individual cases of aggressive prostate cancer in older men, the norm is for the disease to be quite indolent in older men. It is now clear that the treatment of prostate cancer is very different in 50–60 year old men than it is in 90 year men.

Subclinical hypothyroidism is often diagnosed in older adults with a TSH between 5.0 and 10.0 and is typically felt to require treatment with thyroid replacement medications. A study from the Netherlands, as well as other recent data, suggest that aggressive treatment of subclinical hypothyroidism may be harmful in the very elderly [21].

Older individuals have a higher incidence of osteoporosis and vertebral compression fractures. The treatment of vertebral compression fractures with a procedure known as vertebroplasty has not been shown to be appreciably better than a sham procedure [22]. Still, it is not uncommon today for an elderly individual to be whisked from the emergency room into the operating room for a vertebroplasty or kyphoplasty. Discussion of any aggressive treatment of older people requiring acute hospitalization must also consider the increased risk of complications that can occur due to hospitalization [23].

Epidemiologic studies have shown that systolic blood pressure of those in their 80s and 90s tend to be higher [24]. Is this bad? The literature in this population is quite limited. In fact, many elderly patients continue to be treated very aggressively for hypertension despite the fact that the HYVET study only supports a goal systolic blood pressure of 150 [25]. The cost of multiple medications, often bringing down the blood pressure to below 120, and the potential side effects of these medications call into question this standard approach to treatment. The most recent guidelines for the treatment of hypertension recognize these findings, but do not highlight them, making it unlikely that this knowledge will quickly work its way into clinical practice [26].

There is growing evidence regarding the complexity of managing diabetes mellitus in older individuals [27]. Controlling blood sugars too tightly may lead to hypoglycemia, which can have significant implications in older individuals. Long term risks carry a different meaning depending on the life expectancy of the individual. The management of diabetes mellitus in a 90 year old may be significantly different than that of a 50 year old.

A multibillion dollar industry of atypical antipsychotics has recently been called into question by the Office of Inspector General (OIG) [28]. This investigation reflects a number of issues that relate to the medical treatment of the elderly. These very powerful and potentially dangerous medications are typically used off label as a chemical restraint in the management of cognitively impaired elderly patients [29]. There is clearly a huge lack of adequate education of health care professionals as it relates to the treatment and management of dementia, in particular, Alzheimer's disease [30].

These are but a few of the examples of how the care of older people differs and how geriatric medicine may differ from classic internal medicine in ways that go beyond the practical issues of managing chronic illness. That said, there is also a growing amount of evidence that managing chronic illness not only requires clinical acumen (and evidence, which is presently lacking), but new systems of care, in particular, some form of care coordination. In fact, the issue of care coordination is of profound importance as it relates to the training of the healthcare workforce. Geriatricians must have a skill set that allows them to work effectively in a team environment. This requires both leadership and management skills for which physicians rarely receive training. Furthermore, with the financial implications of the growing older population on Medicare and health care costs in the United States, there is also a need for geriatricians to have the expertise to actively participate in policy and program development as new models of care are proposed and implemented [15].

With the aging of the U.S. population, it is still puzzling that there has not been a more robust development of geriatric medicine. What happened? Federal support of GME was supposed to assure an adequate supply of physicians for the Medicare program, but it is well known that many physicians today do not accept new

Medicare patients. Other physicians limit the percentage of Medicare patients in their practice. While recent literature suggests that Medicare patients have access to physicians, this is predominantly due to access to specialists. A recent study still showed that close to 30 % of Medicare beneficiaries have difficulty accessing a primary care physician [31]. The decline in primary care physicians has also been well documented [32]. In regards to the emphasis on specialization, it could be theorized that government financing of GME has made it easier for young physicians to advance directly into subspecialty programs. Prior to 1965 many physicians went into primary care practice prior to deciding whether to subspecialize. An unintended consequence of governmental support of medical education could be that it has limited the free market development of not only geriatrics, but primary care in general, while actually encouraging physicians to go into higher paying subspecialties. With better financial support throughout internship and residency, young doctors do not feel the financial need to enter the marketplace as primary care providers when they can continue on in fellowship programs that lead to much higher incomes. Combining these incentives with those previously mentioned within the realm of GME financing, the decline in both geriatrics and primary care is not surprising.

At the present time, there are over 22,000 physicians board certified in cardiology and close to 7,000 board certified in geriatric medicine. In 1988 the first certification examination (for an "added qualification" at the time) in geriatric medicine was offered. It was offered to physicians who were board certified in Internal Medicine as well as to physicians who were board certified in family medicine. There were 1,659 internists and 752 family medicine physicians who passed the first examination. The majority of these physicians were practicing physicians who "grandfathered" in [33]. The last time physicians were able to grandfather in to passing the examination was in 1994, when 1,568 internists and 771 family medicine physicians passed the exam. The number of geriatricians in the United States reached close to 8,000 at that time. Today, only physicians who complete a geriatric fellowship are eligible to take the board certification exam. Since 2009, there have not been more than 200 internists and 100 family medicine physicians passing the exam each year [34]. As of 2013, there were 4,972 internists and 2,120 family medicine physicians with a valid board certification in geriatric medicine [35]. These numbers generally have been declining every year, as the number of "grandfathered" physicians retiring from practice exceeds the number of physicians completing their fellowships. It has also recently been noted that there has been a decline in the number of physicians entering geriatric fellowships, with the total number dropping to 251 in December of 2011 [36].

Upon the initiation of a geriatric board certification there was clearly an initial rush to getting certified, as well as early growth in the numbers of physicians completing geriatric fellowships. Unfortunately, while there has continued to be growth in other medical specialities, geriatrics has declined. The subsidization of GME as we have described is only part of the story. The other part has to do with the incentives that physicians have that ultimately influence their educational decisions. While financial support during fellowship has encouraged young doctors to specialize, their ultimate income potential factors into the determination of which field to specialize [37]. It is notable that the birth of geriatric medicine as a board certified specialty coincided with changes in how physician reimbursement was determined. Geriatric medicine is amongst the lowest paying physician specialty. Completing a geriatric fellowship in order to enter the lowest paying field is not a good financial incentive. In fact, geriatricians often earn less with their additional training than a primary care internist or family physician. In 1999 a physician who pursued a 1-year geriatric medicine fellowship stood to lose $7,016 annually, and the completion of a 2-year fellowship translated into a net annual loss of $8,592 [38]. In 2006 a geriatrician's median salary was only 92 % of the median salary for a general internist [39]. The reason is that in most medical practices, geriatricians have historically drawn the most complex and frail patients, which, due to the structure of the coding system, leads to lower volumes of visits and to the lowest reimbursement. They are therefore often seen as being less "productive" than other physicians. Clearly, this level of productivity relates solely to reimbursement. The exception to this situation is when geriatricians are part of an organization that receives financial incentives for reduction in hospital utilization or specialty costs, a cost avoidance goal that geriatricians typically are good at doing.

The income gap between primary care physicians and geriatricians with other specialties has grown significantly in the past 20 years. In 1989, the government decided to try to rein in the growth of health care expenditures by changing the physician reimbursement model. President George Bush signed the Omnibus Budget Reconciliation Act of 1989, enacting a physician payment schedule based on a Resource-Based Relative Value Scale (RBRVS) [40]. The means they chose for determining the coding system was to utilize the American Medical Association's (AMA) codes for physician services and to develop a process by which they would determine how physicians would be reimbursed. The RBRVS replaced the previous usual-and-customary system for pricing physician services and was designed to be based on the actual amount of resources necessary to provide a particular physician service. At the time, the two resources studied for each service were physician work and physician practice expense. CMS later added medical malpractice as a third component [41]. Implicitly missing from these calculations are market based phenomena that relate to supply and demand. Also missing are any evidence or value based criteria.

The theory at the time was clearly to find a process to more effectively determine appropriate physician reimbursement. The process that was put in place was under the direct purview of the AMA. A committee was formed to make recommendations to Medicare, but historically, Medicare (under the umbrella of CMS) follows almost all of the recommendations [41]. The committee that was to make these determinations was called the Relative Value Scale Update Committee (RUC) and it was composed of 29 members.

The RUC essentially determines how physicians are paid to care for Medicare beneficiaries. In retrospect, it does not appear that the makeup of this committee was critically evaluated in respect to the impact it would have on differential reimbursement. From the onset, the committee was made up almost exclusively of specialists. In fact, until very recently, there were no regular members of the committee that were geriatricians. A committee whose purpose was to determine physician reimbursement for the care of Medicare beneficiaries had no members with expertise in geriatric medicine. This recently changed with the addition of two permanent seats on the RUC for primary care, one of those seats belonging specifically to a geriatrician. The fact that there is now 1 member out of 29 with expertise in geriatrics is better, but not very encouraging.

Another interesting confounding factor is that the government pays the AMA royalties for the privilege of using their coding system. These royalties have been noted to exceed 70 million dollars a year [42]. The AMA also brings in millions of dollars in revenue from publications that relate to the entire coding system. It is not entirely clear whether all of these revenues are used solely to maintain the coding system, and in fact, it has been recently noted that the RUC process costs about $7 million annually [41]. The AMA also spends a significant amount of money lobbying congress, most recently averaging lobbying expenditures of almost $20 million a year over the past several years [43]. As Medicare is a federally legislated program, and all changes to the program must be legislated by congress, lobbying has a important place in the process and must be recognized. It would appear that the incentive for the AMA's lobbying is to maintain the status quo as it relates to reimbursement.

Medicare reimbursement has been heavily weighted towards procedures and specialists. The office visit codes typically utilized by primary care physicians and geriatricians are historically the lowest reimbursed codes. The AMA claims that the specialist members of the RUC also utilize these very same codes. What they don't point out is that most specialists bring in the majority of their revenue through the procedure codes they use, not the Evaluation and Management (E&M) codes that they share with primary care and geriatrics. Only recently has there been a move towards recognizing the value of the primary care office codes and an attempt to increase the differential reimbursement. This move is encouraging but may be too little and too late. Furthermore, there has yet to be adequate recognition of the importance and value of work performed in nursing facilities. While it has been well documented that nursing home residents have higher health care utilization, the incentives to bring an educated workforce to the patient have been limited. Homebound seniors and those in assisted living facilities form another group of patients who represent higher utilizers of health care services. While gains were made in 2006 in reimbursement for caring for seniors in assisted living facilities and in their homes, the payment for those codes were reduced in 2007. With the reimbursement model that exists today, it is a small wonder that fewer physicians are going into primary care or geriatrics.

The single most impactful part of the Affordable Care Act (ACA) that affected primary care reimbursement was the Primary Care Incentive Program (PCIP): Through this program, Medicare provides a quarterly incentive payment to augment the Medicare payment for primary care services as authorized by the ACA. The incentive payment is equal to 10 % of the Medicare paid amount for primary care services as defined in the Medicare statute. Those services are: New and established patient office or other outpatient services (CPT 99201–99215); Nursing facility care visits and domiciliary, rest home or homecare plan oversight services (CPT 99304–99340); and Patient home visits (CPT 99341–99350). While this bonus program has clearly been helpful to primary care physicians, it has not been a "game-changer" in the sense of leading to the type of significant increase in reimbursement for primary care physicians or geriatricians that might increase market demand for trainees to enter these fields.

The recent addition of transition CPT codes and the upcoming addition of care coordination codes also opens the door to the potential to encourage care coordination activities in medical practices. Ultimately, the success of adding these codes will be dependent on the impact of their actual revenue production on physician reimbursement. Historically, the success of such codes have been limited by both the difficulty of their use and the perceived risk of increased audits for the use of these codes. There is further discussion regarding these codes in the chapter on care coordination.

The ACA has other items incorporated into it that attempt to address workforce issues. Amongst these are provisions to enhance education and training for physician assistants and advanced practice nurses in primary care, as well as provisions that promote the patient-centered medical home model utilizing multidisciplinary teams that include physician assistants and nurse practitioners.

While the ACA does not directly address the need for additional clinical placement slots for nurses and other professions, it does provide for the redistribution of graduate medical education residency slots. The efficacy of this is questionable due to the reasons that we have already reviewed.

The ACA permits, but did not provide funding for, grants to states to establish a Primary Care Extension Program that engages the state health department, Medicaid and Medicare programs, and colleges and/or universities training primary care providers [44]. The grants would require states to assist in the implementation of patient-centered medical homes; develop learning communities for the dissemination of evidenced-based research; gain support from other programs through a national network of programs; and create a sustainability plan for when federal funds will no longer be available. The Primary Care Extension Program was intended to provide opportunities to help primary care providers (e.g., physicians, physician assistants, and nurses) gain new skills in areas such as preventive medicine, health promotion, chronic disease management, mental health and behavioral health services, evidence-based medicine practices, and evidence informed therapies and techniques.

A Senate report released in January of 2013 calls for a number of changes for medical schools and post-graduate education to help the PCP shortage, including: giving medical schools additional funding if they meet a benchmark goal of a certain number of graduates entering primary care residencies; forcing schools to increase recruitment and training of minorities, who are more likely to practice medicine in underserved communities, and; increasing funding for community health centers and the National Health Service Corps, which pays for the loans of physicians who practice in rural areas [45]. None of these recommendations change the dynamics that have been discussed in this chapter and are unlikely to have a significant impact on the number of primary care physicians in this country. Furthermore, the report does not address the need for effective geriatric education of the primary care workforce.

The other question that must be posed in the context of these issues is regarding the ideal role for geriatricians. This is a significant public policy question. Regardless of the role that geriatricians will play in our future health care landscape, there is no question that our country does not have enough geriatricians to fill all of the necessary roles. Furthermore, while the need for geriatricians will continue to increase, there is presently clear evidence that their numbers are continuing to decline. So, where do geriatricians fit into our healthcare infrastructure today?

There might have been a time when there would have been potential for geriatricians to provide primary care for many seniors. In the relative short term that is theoretically difficult based on the low and declining numbers of geriatricians. That leaves geriatricians with the key role of leader and educator. Primary care physicians and specialists alike must be better educated in the appropriate care of our growing older population. Health care systems, patient-centered medical homes and accountable care organizations should have geriatricians leading the development and implementation of appropriate systems of care. Unfortunately, this has not typically occurred. One might postulate that geriatrician leaders could impact the potential effectiveness of such programs. We can only hope that the marketplace will ultimately respond to this possibility in a positive fashion. Incentives being put forward might help the demand for geriatricians if they are perceived as having the ability to positively impact a practice's ability to achieve specific goals. Hospital utilization is one of the more obvious goals that geriatricians are known to be able to impact [46]. PQRS metrics might also have an impact on the hiring of geriatricians, although the specificity for those metrics in the frail elderly is limited at this time [1].

There is a dramatic solution to the physician workforce issue that combines the present lack of primary care physicians and geriatricians. There is general agreement that we will need an increase in physicians, and primary care physicians in particular, in the coming years [47]. What if we were to find a way to train more primary care geriatricians? As new models of care are developed that promote team based care, it is possible that market forces will begin to attract trainees into primary care, although this may take some time. Since there have been proposals to increase the GME cap on residents, what if the cap were solely raised for primary care geriatrics? The GME Initiative has made such a proposal [48]. One of the concerns about increasing the cap without specificity is that it will ultimately only lead to more physicians becoming specialists. While there might be no guarantee that primary care geriatricians wouldn't go into subspecialties, they would at least move forward with adequate competencies in geriatric medicine. Clearly, another factor that would need to be tied to such a proposal is reimbursement. It is not difficult to foresee an increase in reimbursement to primary care geriatricians as a means to assure an adequate growth in the workforce. An approach such as this would continue to require the development of geriatrician educators and leaders, which would be provided for by the continued growth of geriatric fellowship programs. Indeed, further financial incentives for geriatric fellowship programs would complement this approach. The politics of such a proposal are enormous, but the societal implications of not developing an adequate workforce to appropriately care for Medicare beneficiaries is equally profound. Furthermore, the United States has a history of making dramatic changes in order to deal with major issues, whether it be the New Deal, or the development of the atomic bomb. Our country will just have to decide how important the lack of geriatricians is when it comes to controlling the growth and adding value to a Medicare program that has continued to take up a larger share of the federal budget.

Perhaps a more pragmatic and manageable approach would be to allow geriatric medicine certification to all physicians and to provide enhanced reimbursement for those who are certified. This approach could be simpler and would have the benefit of providing an immediate incentive for the existing workforce of primary care physicians to improve their competencies in geriatric medicine. It would not forestall the continued need for fellowship trained geriatricians as both educators and leaders. Obviously, the continued training of young physicians would require more geriatrician educators. And, as noted before, geriatrician leaders are essential for effectively carrying out large scale programs that rely on the fundamental principles of geriatric medicine. It would still be necessary to increase the incentives for physicians to enter into geriatric fellowship programs, something that might be possible under the existing GME structure. One possibility would be a loan forgiveness program. Increasing slots for geriatric fellows would not work, as the existing fellowship slots don't even come close to being filled. Ultimately, there must be financial incentives attached to doing a geriatric fellowship, otherwise we will not be able to make up for the existing incentives that have driven young physicians away from the field.

A third, and not necessarily separate, approach recognizes that we are presently dealing with inadequate competencies in geriatrics not only in the primary care specialties, but in the medical and surgical subspecialties as well. It would seem logical that all training programs and certification examinations should be structured to focus on achieving a minimum set of geriatric competencies. The Next Accreditation System (NAS) has just begun implementation and will hopefully provide a platform for the introduction of such competencies [49]. The development and implementation of specific milestones provides an excellent opportunity to instill geriatric focused educational goals into all training programs. Perhaps requiring these competencies in order to receive GME funding would result in a more appropriately educated workforce. Whatever the approach, there will be significant political roadblocks to overcome.

Physicians are not the only part of the workforce that needs to be adequately prepared to care for our aging population. Most physicians are trained to work individually. Geriatricians are generally trained for and are used to working in team environments. With that said, every member of the team must be trained to work within a team environment in order for the team to function effectively. There is growing evidence that teams can be trained for improved effectiveness [50]. Nurse practitioners, physician assistants, nurses, social workers, physical therapists, occupational therapists, speech therapists, pharmacists and certified nursing assistants must all be fully trained to appropriately care for our older patients.

According to the Institute of medicine study, "Retooling for an Aging America: Building the Healthcare Workforce," [51] there are serious shortages in all areas of the geriatric healthcare workforce. Less than 1 % of RN's were certified in geriatrics. Only 29 % of baccalaureate programs had a certified faculty member and only one third of the programs even required exposure to geriatrics. Less than 3 % of Advance Practice RN's (APRN's) were certified in geriatrics and only 300 geriatric APRN's were graduating annually. There are only 13 programs for academic geriatric dentistry and geriatrics is not explicitly tested on board examinations. Fewer than 1 % of pharmacists are certified in geriatrics and there are only 10 residency programs in geriatric pharmacy. There are no advance training programs in geriatrics for physician assistants and fewer than 1 % specialize in geriatrics. Despite the fact that the NIA estimated a need for 70,000 geriatric social workers by 2020, only 4 % of social workers specialize in geriatrics. 40 % of schools for social work lack faculty in aging and 80 % of BSW programs have no coursework in aging. Only 29 % of MSW programs offer a focus on aging. The national EMT curriculum does not have a module for geriatrics. Only 22 % of undergraduate dietetics and nutrition programs offer courses in aging. Despite the large number of medicare beneficiaries that see a podiatrist, only one of eight schools of podiatric medicine lists a course devoted to geriatrics.

There have been efforts in recent years to increase the training opportunities for all health care professionals. The Medicare program, for example, not only supports the training of residents but has made some payments to hospitals for its share of the direct costs of nursing and allied health training programs. In 2001 Congress introduced the All Payer Graduate Medical Education Act [50], which would collect additional GME funds through a 1 % tax on private health plans. Part of this revenue was directed toward the graduate education of "non-physician health professionals" [52]. The Nurse Education, Expansion, and Development Act [50] proposes to provide grants to nursing schools, in part, to develop "post-baccalaureate residency programs to prepare nurses for practice in specialty areas where nursing shortages are more severe." These measures are for the training of health professionals in general, however, and do not necessarily support advanced geriatric training [53].

The healthcare workforce issues clearly go far beyond the training of physicians and the number of geriatricians. At the end of the day, however, physicians are the ultimate driver of health care costs as they are the key decision makers for the care decisions that drive health care expenditures. This brings us back to the question of what can be done to increase the number of geriatricians in this country. We have previously suggested changes to both the certification process and the reimbursement system. However, this doesn't get to the issue of whether a medical student even develops an interest in geriatrics. Unfortunately, it appears that most medical students start school with little interest in geriatrics [54]. The irony of this fact is that geriatricians tend to have the highest job satisfaction across a variety of specialties [55]. The issue clearly becomes one of directing trainees into geriatrics.

What makes a medical student choose a career in geriatrics? Typically, medical students determine the direction of their training during their third year of medical school. They must make their residency choice during their fourth year of medical school. This gives very limited opportunities for students to be exposed to geriatrics. There are very few required rotations in geriatrics, and third year medical student rotations are typically made up of required rotations. Elective rotations are usually taken during the fourth year, often after students have made their residency program decision.

What type of experiences do students presently have when it comes to geriatrics? The first major issue is that of the negative stereotypes that students encounter prior to and during their training. Third year medical students typically see older patients at their worst, in the acute hospital setting. Many of the patients that they see have physical and cognitive disabilities [56]. Students in various fields typically see working with seniors as being depressing, and tend to rank geriatrics near the bottom [57]. What can be done to change this? Early exposure to healthier older adults has been shown to have a positive impact on the interest in students in going into geriatrics [58]. One effective strategy for providing students with a positive experience is pairing them with older adults who act as mentors [59]. In an intriguing finding, and one that recognizes the need for incentives to encourage positive exposure opportunities, Cummings found that 60 % of social work students would have an interest in a geriatric experience if a stipend was included [60]. Medical students are certainly influenced by their professors and attending physicians [61]. It is clearly important to expose students to physician mentors who can demonstrate the positive aspects of geriatric care [62]. The obvious problem with this approach is the limited number of such mentors at the present time. As we train geriatricians, we need to focus on training them to be effective role models.

The existing structure of medical school training, GME subsidies and reimbursement incentives puts us in a difficult "chicken and egg" situation. We have a scarcity of positive physician role models to provide mentoring to students in their early years. The present educational structure typically exposes students to older adults at their worst. Subsidies give residents the opportunity to choose specialties where the existing reimbursement structure provides a financial incentive. Most recommendations for changing this have been of the "incremental" type and seem to be doomed to failure before they even start. One could argue that we need major game changing approaches that allow students to obtain positive experiences while setting up the necessary economic incentives to encourage them to consider a career in the field of geriatric medicine. This is certainly not limited to medical students, but that is ultimately where the greatest impact on the delivery of health care will occur. Furthermore, once more physicians begin to choose careers in geriatrics, nurses and other allied health professionals will certainly follow.

To summarize, geriatric medicine is a uniquely different specialty that recognizes the differences in the clinical management of older adults. Faced with a Medicare program whose costs have risen dramatically, and a workforce that is incentivized to deliver unproven and costly care, it seems obvious that we must not only stem the decline in geriatricians, but increase their numbers dramatically.

Furthermore, it is imperative that the education of all physicians, as well as other health care professionals, be altered to bring about improved competencies in the care of older adults. The existing GME structure is inadequate in achieving this goal, as is the present system of reimbursement. Small incremental changes will not have a significant impact on the present situation. Dramatic changes must be made in order to bring about a workforce that can deliver appropriate care to our growing older population.

References

1. Cooper RA. It's time to address the problem of physician shortages: graduate medical education is the key. Ann Surg. 2007;246(4):527–34.
2. Grumbach K. Fighting hand to hand over physician workforce policy. Health Aff. 2002; 21(5):13–27.
3. Baker JP. Reinventing a specialty: how pediatrics survived its own success. Pediatrics. 1998; 102(1):197–200.
4. The American Board of Pediatrics. Workforce Data 2013–2014. https://www.abp.org/abpwebsite/stats/wrkfrc/workforcebook.pdf
5. Fried LP, Hall WJ. Leading on behalf of an aging society. J Am Geriatr Soc. 2008;56: 1791–5.
6. Rich EC, Liebow M, Srinivasan M. Medicare financing of graduate medical education. JGIM. 2002;17:283–92.
7. Twenty-first report of COGME, improving value in graduate medical education, Aug 2013.
8. Pugno PA, Gillanders WR, Kozakowski SM. The direct, indirect, and intangible benefits of graduate medical education programs to their sponsoring institutions and communities. J Grad Med Educ. 2010;2(2):154–9.
9. Brubaker JK. The birth of a new specialty: geriatrics. J Lanc Gen Hosp. Fall 2008;3(3): 105–7.
10. Leipzig RN, Granville L, Simpson D, et al. Keeping granny safe on July 1: a consensus on minimum geriatrics competencies for graduating medical students. Acad Med. 2009;84(5): 604–10.
11. Monette M, Hill A. Arm-twisting medical schools for core geriatric training. CMAJ. 2012;184(10):E515–6.
12. History of Mount Sinai's geriatric medicine. http://www.mountsinai.org/patient-care/service-areas/geriatrics-and-aging/about-us/history
13. Forciea MA. Geriatric medicine: a brief history. UPHS; 2012. http://www.med.upenn.edu/gec/user_documents/Forciea-HistoryofGeriMedicine.pdf
14. Wasserman MR, Holthaus KM. KCosgrove, TheMedWiseCenter–an innovation in primary care geriatrics. Continuum. 1998;18(1):18–23.
15. Boult C, Counsell SR, Leipzig RM. The urgency of preparing primary care physicians to care for older people with chronic illnesses. Health Aff. 2010;29(5):811–9.
16. Inouye SK, Studenski S, Tinetti ME, Kuchel GA. Geriatric syndromes: clinical research and policy implications of a core geriatric concept. J Am Geriatric Soc. 2007;55(5):780–91.
17. Flaherty JH, Morley JE, Murphy DJ, Wasserman MR. The development of outpatient Clinical Glidepaths. J Am Geriatr Soc. 2002;50(11):1886–901.
18. Yoshikawa T. Future direction of geriatrics: gerogeriatrics. J Am Geriatr Soc. 2012;60(4): 632–4.
19. The Atrial Fibrillation Follow-up Investigation of Rhythm Management (AFFIRM) Investigators. A comparison of rate control and rhythm control in patients with atrial fibrillation. NEJM. 2002;347:1825–33.

20. Stangelberger A, Waldert M, Djavan B. Prostate cancer in elderly men. Rev Urol. 2008;10(2):111–9. Spring.
21. Meneilly GS. Should subclinical hypothyroidism in elderly patients be treated. CMAJ. 2005;172(5):633.
22. Buchbinder R, Osborne RH, Ebeling PR, et al. A randomized trial of vertebroplasty for painful osteoporotic vertebral fractures. NEJM. 2009;361(6):557–68.
23. Walsh KA, Bruza JM. Hospitalization of the elderly. Ann Long Term Care. 2007;15(11).
24. Goodwin JS. Embracing complexity: a consideration of hypertension in the very old. J Gerontol. 2003;58A(7):653–8.
25. HYVET, Hypertension in the very elderly trial. http://www.hyvet.com/general/Hyvet.asp
26. James PA, Oparil S, Carter BL, et al. 2014 evidence-based guideline for the management of high blood pressure in adults: report from the panel members appointed to the eighth joint national committee (JNC 8). JAMA. 2014;311(5):507–20.
27. Kirkman MS, Briscoe VJ, Clark N, et al. Diabetes in older adults: a consensus report. J Am Geriatr Soc. 2012;60(12):2342–56.
28. Office of Inspector General. Report (OEI-07-08-00150) medicare atypical antipsychotic drug claims for elderly nursing home residents. http://oig.hhs.gov/oei/reports/oei-07-08-00150.asp
29. Lindsey PL. Psychotropic medication use among older adults: what all nurses need to know. J Gerontol Nurs. 2009;35(9):28–38.
30. Reuben D, Levin J, Wenger N. Closing the dementia care gap: can referral to the Alzheimer's Association chapters help? Alzheimers Dement. 2009;5(6):498–502.
31. Shartzer A, Zuckerman R, McDowell A, Kronick R. Access to physicians' services for medicare beneficiaries. ASPE Issue Brief, 22 Aug 2013.
32. Chen C, Petterson S, Phillips RL, et al. Toward graduate medical education (GME) accountability: measuring the outcomes of GME institutions. Acad Med. 2013;88(9):1267–80.
33. Geriatric medicine training and practice in the United States at the beginning of the 21st century. ADGAP. 2002. http://www.americangeriatrics.org/files/documents/gwps/ADGAP%20Full%20Report.pdf
34. http://www.abim.org/pdf/data-candidates-certified/Number-Certified-Annually.pdf
35. http://www.abim.org/pdf/data-candidates-certified/all-candidates.pdf
36. Chris Langston, Health AGEnda, The John A. Hartford Foundation. 2012. http://www.jhartfound.org/blog/decline-in-geriatric-fellows-defies-pay-boost-10-10/
37. Phillips RL, Dodoo MS, Petterson S, et al. What influences medical student & resident choices? The Robert Graham center: policy studies in family medicine and primary care. 2009. http://www.graham-center.org/online/graham/home/publications/onepagers/2010/op67-income-disparities.html
38. Weeks WB, Wallace AE. Return on educational investment in geriatrics training. J Am Geriatri Soc. 2004;52(11):1940–5.
39. Association of Directors of Geriatric Academic Programs (ADGAP). The Status of Geriatrics Workforce Study, Training & Practice Update. 2008;6(1):1–7.
40. Blasier RD, Twetten M. Understanding the RUC. http://www.aaos.org/news/aaosnow/jun11/advocacy2.asp
41. Eaton J, Center For Public Integrity. Little-known AMA group has big influence on medicare payments. Kaiser Health News. 27 Oct 2010.
42. Roy A. Why the American medical association had 72 million reasons to shrink doctors' pay. Forbes, 28 Nov 2011.
43. http://www.opensecrets.org/lobby/clientsum.php?id=D000000068
44. Phillips Jr RL, Kaufman A, Mold JW, et al. The primary care extension program: a catalyst for change. Ann Fam Med. 2013;11(2):173–8.
45. Pittman D. RUC targeted at senate hearing on primary care. Washington Correspondent, MedPage Today, 29 Jan 2013.
46. Fenton JJ, Levine MD, Mahoney LD, Heagerty PJ, Wagner EH. Bringing geriatricians to the front lines: evaluation of a quality improvement intervention in primary care. J Am Board Fam Med. 2006;19(4):331–9.

47. Voorhees KI, Prado-Gutierrez A, Epperly T, Derksen D. A proposal for reform of the structure and financing of primary care graduate medical education. Fam Med. 2013;45(3):164–70.
48. Nasca TJ, Philibert I, Brigham T, Flynn TC. The next GME accreditation system. NEJM. 2012;366:1051–6.
49. Salas E, DiazGranados D, Klein C, et al. Does team training improve team performance? A meta-analysis. Hum Factors. 2008;50:903–33.
50. Institute of Medicine. Retooling for an aging America: building the healthcare workforce. Washington, DC: The National Academies Press; 2008.
51. All Payer Graduate Medical Education Act of 00. HR 2178. 107th congress. 14 June 2001.
52. Nurse Education, Expansion, and Development Act of 00. S 446. 110th congress, 1st session. 31 Jan 2007.
53. Fitzgerald JT, Wray LA, Halter JB, Williams BC. Relating medical students' knowledge, attitudes, and experience to an interest in geriatric medicine. Gerontologist. 2003;43(6):849–55.
54. Krout JA, McKernan P. The impact of gerontology inclusion on 12th grade student perceptions of aging, older adults and working with elders. Gerontol Geriatr Educ. 2007;27(4):23–40.
55. Leigh JP, Kravitz RL, Schembri M, et al. Physician career satisfaction across specialties. Arch Intern Med. 2002;162:1577–84.
56. Cummings SM, Galambos C. Predictors of graduate social work students' interest in aging-related work. J Gerontol Soc Work. 2003;39(3):77–94.
57. Bernard MA, McAuley WJ, Belzer JA, Neal KS. An evaluation of a low-intensity intervention to introduce medical students to healthy older people. J Am Geriatr Soc. 2003;51(3):419–23.
58. Westmoreland GR, Counsell SR, Sennour Y. Improving medical student attitudes toward older patients through a "council of elders" and reflective writing experience. J Am Geriatr Soc. 2009;57(2):315–20.
59. Cummings SM, Adler G, DeCoster VA. Factors influencing graduate-social-work students' interest in working with elders. Educ Gerontol. 2005;31(8):643–55.
60. Haidet P, Stein HF. The role of the student-teacher relationship in the formation of physicians. The hidden curriculum as process. J Gen Intern Med. 2006;21 Suppl 1:S16–20.
61. Hazzard WR. Mentoring across the professional lifespan in academic geriatrics. J Am Geriatr Soc. 1999;47(12):1466–70.
62. Wright SM, Kern DE, Kolodner K, et al. Attributes of excellent attending physician role models. NEJM. 1998;339:1986–93.

Chapter 7
Medicare and Medicaid Coordination: Special Case of the Dual Eligible Beneficiary

Gregg Warshaw and Peter A. DeGolia

Background

The Affordable Care Act of 2010 (ACA) includes several provisions related to the cost and quality of the care received by dually eligible Medicare and Medicaid beneficiaries. The "dual eligibles" are low income older adults and younger persons with significant disabilities. More than nine million Medicare beneficiaries are also enrolled in the Medicaid program. Sixty percent are age 65 years and older and 40 % are under age 65 [1]. Among the participants in Medicare and Medicaid, the dual eligible population includes many recipients who have the lowest incomes and highest chronic disease burden. It is recognized that providing care for the dual eligible population is an expensive component of both the Medicaid and Medicare budgets. The "Duals" comprise only 15 % of total Medicaid enrollment yet represent 39 % of annual Medicaid expenditures. Similarly for Medicare, duals represent 21 % of Medicare enrollees but 36 % of Medicare expenditures [2]. In 2007, Medicare, Medicaid, supplemental insurance, and out-of- pocket expenses, on

G. Warshaw, M.D. (✉)
Geriatric Medicine Program and Department of Family and Community Medicine, College of Medicine, University of Cincinnati, 231 Albert Sabin Way, PO Box 670504, Cincinnati, OH 45267-0504, USA
e-mail: gregg.warshaw@uc.edu

P.A. DeGolia, M.D.
Department of Family Medicine, University Hospitals Case Medical Center, 11100 Euclid Ave, Cleveland, OH 44106, USA

average, amounted to $28,500 per dual-eligible beneficiary; nearly twice as much as for other Medicare beneficiaries [3]. Since the costs of Medicaid are shared between the federal government and the states; Congress and state legislatures are seeking more effective and less costly approaches to caring for the "Duals" population.

"Duals" Illness Burden and Diversity

One of the challenges for health planners seeking strategies to improve the care experience and outcomes for the dual eligibles is that the population is very diverse. Many of the older "duals" live in nursing homes and suffer from chronic illnesses, such, as, Alzheimer's disease. Among the older adults living in the community, functional impairment is common, although some older "duals" in the community are independent and healthy. The remainder of the beneficiaries are younger adults with mental or physical disabilities. Eligibility for Medicare for these younger adults comes through the social security disability system (generally eligible after 24 months on Social Security Disability benefits) or by eligibility for certain end-stage renal disease services (renal dialysis or transplant). In summary, 43 % of all Dual beneficiaries have at least one mental or cognitive impairment; while 60 % have multiple chronic conditions. Nineteen percent live in institutional settings, compared to only 3 % of non-dual eligible Medicare beneficiaries [4].

Care Coordination Challenges

Qualifying for both Medicare and Medicaid reduces the out-of-pocket cost burden for dual eligible beneficiaries. However, many dual-eligible patients and their caregivers experience difficulties navigating the health care system. The division of responsibility across the Medicare and Medicaid programs only intensifies these problems for dual eligibles. For example, many physicians who care for Medicare beneficiaries may not be familiar with the benefits and services available through Medicaid. Also, poorly aligned financial incentives may discourage health care providers and the Medicare and Medicaid programs from coordinating care, leading to costly and inefficient care.

In general, Medicare will reimburse acute care and physician visits, and Medicaid will be the primary payer for community based long-term services and supports. Because of the separate financing streams and conflicting incentives, Medicare and Medicaid cannot realize equal savings from their investment in improved care. For example, patients may be moved from a nursing home where Medicaid is the primary payer, to a hospital, where Medicare is the primary payer, to shift costs from one program to the other. Better long-term care coordination, for example, may result in reduced hospitalizations, but these saving may benefit the Medicare program far more than the Medicaid program. These inefficiencies, relatively poor care coordination, and combined with the high costs of care are driving the need for change on how the care for the "duals" is organized [4, 5].

Models of Care Prior to the ACA

Legal statute mandates Medicare and Medicaid. These mandates are significantly different. The Social Security Act [6] mandates that Medicare cover services that are medically "reasonable and necessary for the diagnosis or treatment of illness or injury or to improve the functioning of a malformed body member". Consequently, this coverage tends to be focused toward acute care services. Medicaid, on the other hand, pays for "necessary medical services and …rehabilitation and other services to help …individuals attain or retain capability for independence or self-care" [7]. The Medicaid program's benefits are more focused on the care of chronic disease.

Medicare is the primary insurer for dual eligibles and covers services such as physician, hospital, hospice, skilled nursing facility, home health services and durable medical equipment. Since the passage of the Medicare Part D program in 2006, Medicare also covers prescription medications.

Medicaid is organized as 50 state programs each having their own rules and processes for determining eligibility for benefits, approved services, and payments. These programs include both managed care and fee-for-service models. Some states allow potential Medicaid beneficiaries with higher income and asset levels to qualify if they are "medically needy" and have high health care bills. Qualifying for Medicaid coverage is affected by a person's income and assets as well as individual state coverage and payment policies. Medicaid generally covers services not provided by Medicare. These services include long-term care services such as custodial nursing facility care, home and community-based services (e.g. personal care, social service assistance), dental, vision, and transportation. Approximately two-thirds of the Medicaid benefit package is offered at the option of the state [8], resulting in significant geographic variation in coverage. This variation can apply to dental, vision, and therapy services, as well as the amount of hospital coverage. As state budgetary problems mount, pressure to restrict or reduce Medicaid services result. For example, in 2004 seven states reduced dental and chiropractic services while five states restricted podiatric, psychological services, therapy services and mental health therapies [9].

Medicare has coverage gaps and that often requires cost sharing for covered benefits. Medicaid helps fill many gaps for dual eligible beneficiaries. State Medicaid programs are not required to pay the full cost-sharing amount that Medicare pays as long as their payment policies are written into their state plan [8]. Consequently, certain services may be reimbursed at a lower rate or not at all. When Medicare cost sharing and benefits change, such as limitations on home health services, the cost of one program is shifted to the other and impacts access to care and quality of care for dual eligible beneficiaries.

Medicare Advantage

Prior to the passage of the Affordable Care Act of 2010, the vast majority of dual eligible beneficiaries were enrolled in fee-for-service coverage. An alternative care model option for Medicare beneficiaries is managed care. This option has been available to Medicare beneficiaries since the 1970s. Originally developed as "Medicare+Choice" plans, Medicare beneficiaries were offered the option of enrolling in private health plans for their benefits. With passage of the Medicare Modernization Act of 2003, Congress replaced Medicare+Choice with Medicare Advantage which expanded the types of managed care models to choose from and increased payments to insurance companies to encourage participation [10].

Medicare Advantage plans are generally offered by health insurance companies or large provider organizations. These plans include health maintenance organizations, preferred provider organizations, private fee-for-service plans, or special needs plans. Medicare beneficiaries cannot be mandated to enroll in managed care plans as federal law provides for "freedom of choice". States can mandate Medicaid beneficiaries to enroll in Medicaid managed care plans but this does not apply to dual eligibles. These beneficiaries are considered to be Medicare beneficiaries first.

Over 14 million beneficiaries (28 % of the Medicare population) enrolled in a Medicare Advantage plan in 2013. Enrollment is concentrated in urban areas and varies widely across the states with 42 % of Medicare beneficiaries enrolled in Oregon, and only 3 % in Wyoming. Two-thirds of beneficiaries chose an HMO model plan [11].

Special Needs Plans (A Form of Medicare Advantage)

Special Needs Plans (SNPs) were authorized by Congress in 2003 to focus on specific subtypes of dual eligible beneficiaries with the intent to integrate the financing and delivery of care for the full range of health care needs. This averts some of the coordination–of-benefit problems faced in fee-for-service or non-integrated managed care programs. Integrated care delivery is intended to align financing with incentives to achieve better care coordination and quality of care.

These plans were developed on the assumption that improved quality of care would reduce potentially avoidable emergency department visits, hospitalizations, and nursing facility admissions while saving Medicare funds [12]. Enrollment in a SNP does not necessarily mean a dual eligible beneficiary will receive integrated care. These plans can manage just the Medicare benefits but have the potential to coordinate Medicare benefits with state-administered Medicaid benefits. There are D-SNP (dual eligible SNP), I-SNP (Institutional, usually nursing home based, SNP), and C-SNP (Chronic disease SNP) programs. D-SNPs account for 82 % of all SNP enrollees, although, nationwide, in 2013, only 12 % of dual-eligible beneficiaries were in D-SNPs [11].

One SNP model of care that integrates Medicare and Medicaid services is based on a voluntary integration approach. Minnesota Senior Health Options, a capitated model, started in 1997 and Massachusetts Senior Care Options begun in 2004 are examples of voluntary integrated programs where dual-eligible beneficiaries choose to enroll in a SNP for their Medicare benefits and voluntarily enroll in the same health plan which has contracted with the state Medicaid agency to manage their Medicaid benefits. The state oversees a single contract with participating plans that provide Medicare and Medicaid services through a capitated system with payments combined at the plan level rather than the state level. This approach minimizes regulatory duplication and differences between Medicare and Medicaid while streamlining processes such as enrollment, grievances, and data reporting.

A second SNP model of care has dual eligibles required to enroll in a capitated Medicaid managed care program administered by a managed care organization while allowing the individual to choose whether or not to participate in a capitated Medicare program, a Managed Fee-for-Service Model (MFFS). This model has been implemented in Arizona and Texas [13].

These models were the prototypes for the ACA Financial Alignment Demonstrations, and the states are modifying their approach to dual eligibles based on these early experiences (see below).

State Demonstration Waiver Programs

Medicare granted waiver status for several states to implement State Demonstration Waiver programs to promote the alignment of finances and service with outcomes for dually eligible beneficiaries prior to the passage of the Affordable Care Act. The Minnesota Senior Health Options and Disability Health Options program and Massachusetts Senior Care Options began as waiver programs. The Wisconsin Partnership Program involves community-based organizations entering into a Medicaid managed care contract with the Wisconsin Department of Health and Family Services and a Medicare contract with CMS. The community agencies are responsible for all participant services and receive a monthly capitated payment. This program serves nursing facility certified physically disabled dual eligibles and seniors over 55 years of age [14].

The Program of All-Inclusive Care for the Elderly

The Program of All-Inclusive Care for the Elderly (PACE) stands out as a successful example of a seamlessly integrated program that brings together Medicare and Medicaid benefits into one delivery system. Dual eligible beneficiaries are the majority of enrollees in these programs. As of February, 2014, there are 100 PACE programs operating in 31 states [15]. PACE programs tend to be small and personal, serving nursing home-eligible individuals 55 years of age or older who live in the community served by the PACE organization. Individuals managed within these programs are primarily community-dwelling but also include participants who transition to custodial care in nursing facilities. Interdisciplinary team-based care directs this comprehensive medical and social delivery program which offers adult day health center services, transportation, in-home and referral services based on individual needs (see Box 7.1 for a PACE client case example).

> **Box 7.1 Case Example: The Program of All-Inclusive Care for the Elderly**
> G.O. is a 72 year old Woman with advanced Alzheimer's type dementia with behavioral problems. Historically she was combative and resistant to care; often refusing to take her prescribed medications. She qualified for Long Term Care Services and Support through a community-based agency which provided her 32 h per week of home health aide services and a social service case worker. She frequently was admitted to the local hospital following acute changes in mental status, often associated with urinary tract infections or dehydration. Her medical care was limited as it was difficult to transport her to her primary care physician's office and her behavior became unmanageable while at the office. Her primary care physician expressed frustration in trying to manage her care as he did not see her in the office and was often responding to crises and completing paper work to authorize specific services. He felt disconnected from her care. Her family was committed to caring for her at home, but G.O.'s care needs and frequent medical problems caused significant caregiver strain. This led to custodial care placement following an acute illness in which G.O. was hospitalized.
>
> After a month in a long-term care facility, a family member discovered the local PACE program. Mrs. O's family decided to make a second attempt at keeping her at home. Upon enrollment in the PACE program, G.O. attended the PACE Center (an adult day health center) 5 days a week. She received special care and activities designed to meet her social and health care needs. While at the PACE Center she would be evaluated by medical, nursing, social work, and dietary staff. Modifications in her medication regimen were made. The PACE health professionals worked with G.O.'s family to address care needs at home and assist them in managing her medical regimen. Intermittent respite stays were organized to give the family necessary relief from day-to-day caregiving. Today, 2 years after enrolling in the PACE program, G.O. has not been hospitalized in over a year, continues to live at home with family, and attends the PACE program regularly.

Most PACE programs employ staff providers. However, some employ community physicians, often with PACE advance practice registered nurses assisting in the management of their panel of participants. In one PACE program in the Midwest, community-based primary care physicians are expected to participate once a month in a conference call to the interdisciplinary team (IDT) during regular IDT meetings to review all of the participants managed by the physician. Care plans are reviewed and developed after each 6-month comprehensive assessment. Physicians are paid for their involvement in these care coordination activities. Community providers must have unrestricted appointments for continuity of care and provide 24 h call coverage.

PACE programs are capitated and reimbursement rates are tied to a frailty adjuster based on limitation in Activities of Daily Living. PACE plans negotiate a Medicaid rate with their state Medicaid organization and must provide services through a contracted network of collaborating agencies. CMS has evaluated PACE programs and found that they have positive sustainable outcomes for reduced hospitalizations, improved health status and quality of life, and lower mortality rates compared to similar non-PACE cohorts [16].

Lessons from Previous Demonstration Projects

Lessons from previous demonstration projects targeted at improving the care of the "duals" population help to define some of the characteristics of successful, integrated, well-coordinated, less costly approach to care for this complex population [17–19].

- Many adults in the dual-beneficiary population have multiple chronic illnesses or significant mental health illness that requires intensive care coordination. This may include care managers attending clinical appointments, keeping track of upcoming appointments, making home visits, making telephone contact, etc.
- Care coordinators need to be able to work comfortably across the spectrum of acute and community- based long-term services and supports (CB-LTSS) services. Ideally, care coordination is provided by one individual who has a full grasp of the resources commonly utilized by the "duals" population. Ongoing education for the care managers is essential.
- Access to behavioral health care remains limited in many communities and is critical to well being, particularly for the younger "duals" with significant mental health illness.
- Functional limitations (e.g., inability to leave one's home without assistance), and limited transportation to medical services interferes with access to medical visits and lowers the quality of care.
- States with low Medicaid reimbursement rates are experiencing difficulty attracting managed care organizations to participate in capitated dual eligible demonstrations

ACA Provisions Directly Related to the Care of the Duals

The Centers for Medicare and Medicaid Services (CMS) administers the Medicare and Medicaid programs, which provide health care to almost one in every three Americans. CMS directly employs over 4,500 employees, sub-contracts with many others, and has an annual budget well over $800 billion. The Center for Medicare and the Center for Medicaid and CHIP (Children's Health Insurance Program) Services have traditionally been separate CMS entities with limited coordination of effort. In response to the challenges facing the dual eligible population, the ACA established the Federal Coordinated Health Care Office (FCHCO or Duals Office). The goals of this small office are [20]:

- Providing dual eligible beneficiaries full access to the benefits to which such individuals are entitled to under the Medicare and Medicaid programs.
- Simplifying the processes for dual eligible beneficiaries to access the items and services they are entitled to under the Medicare and Medicaid programs.
- Improving the quality of health care and long-term services for dual eligible beneficiaries.
- Increasing dual eligible beneficiaries understanding of and satisfaction with coverage under the Medicare and Medicaid programs.
- Eliminating regulatory conflicts between rules under the Medicare and Medicaid programs.
- Improving care continuity and ensuring safe and effective care transitions for dual eligible beneficiaries.
- Eliminating cost-shifting between the Medicare and Medicaid program and among related health care providers.
- Improving the quality of performance of providers of services and suppliers under the Medicare and Medicaid programs.

In addition to the Dual's Office, the ACA also established the Center for Medicare and Medicaid Innovation (CMMI). The ACA provides CMMI with significant budget authority to test and expand innovative models of care, including models involving dual eligibles. A number of other provisions in the ACA effect the care provided to dual eligible beneficiaries and these are summarized in Table 7.1.

Financial Alignment Demonstrations

In 2011, the Duals Office began the Medicare-Medicaid Financial Alignment Demonstration. The program allows state Medicaid offices to develop innovative approaches to improve the coordination of care for the dual eligible population, while adding efficiencies and incentives that will reduce the cost of care. Initially, 15 states were awarded $1 million planning awards (California, Colorado, Connecticut, Massachusetts, Michigan, Minnesota, New York, North Carolina, Oklahoma, Oregon, South Carolina, Tennessee, Vermont, Washington and Wisconsin). Subsequently, several states have submitted specific proposals to CMS that allows for an integration of Medicaid and Medicare dollars [22]. These financial alignment demonstrations can take two forms:

- **Capitated Model:** A State, CMS, and a health plan enter into a three-way contract, and the plan receives a prospective blended payment to provide comprehensive, coordinated care.
- **Managed Fee-for-Service Model:** A State and CMS enter into an agreement by which the State would be eligible to benefit from savings resulting from initiatives designed to improve quality and reduce costs for both Medicare and Medicaid.

Table 7.1 Affordable care act provisions relating to the care of dually eligible Medicare and Medicaid beneficiaries

New CMS offices/centers
Federal Coordinated Health Care Office to improve coordination of care for dual eligibles (FCHCO or Duals Office)
Center for Medicare and Medicaid Innovation to test new models of care (CMMI or Innovation Center)
Coordination of care
Independence at home Medicare demonstration project for beneficiaries with chronic illness
Medicaid option to provide health homes for beneficiaries with chronic conditions
Medicaid waivers involving dual eligibles
Preventive benefits (provisions not exclusive to dual eligibles)
New Medicare annual wellness benefit
Medicare and Medicaid preventive services
Medicare part D prescription drug plans
Improved calculation of Low-Income Subsidy (LIS) benchmark premium
Elimination of cost-sharing for certain full benefit dual eligible beneficiaries
Dispensing techniques for medicines prescribed for long-term care facility residents
Inspector General studies of Part D plan formularies
Medication therapy management programs (MTMP) for at-risk enrollees
Medicare advantage plans
Extends the authority for MA plans for special needs individuals (SNP)
Permanently authorized the senior housing facility demonstration
Hold harmless for Program for All-Inclusive Care for the Elderly (PACE)
Long-term care (provisions not exclusive to dual eligibles)
Medicaid community first choice option
Money follows the person demonstration extended
Temporary spousal impoverishment protection
Advisory bodies
Medicaid and CHIP Payment and Access Commission (MACPAC) to study the interaction of Medicaid and Medicare policies
Independent Payment Advisory Board (IPAB) to take into account the unique needs of dual eligibles

Adapted by the author based on: The Henry J. Kaiser Family Foundation's [21]

The State proposals are reviewed by CMS and then a Memorandum of Understanding (MUO) is signed between CMS and the State. At the start of 2014, eight States had completed signed MUO's with CMS, most pursuing the capitated model (California, Illinois, Massachusetts, Ohio, New York, South Carolina, Virginia, and Washington), Minnesota completed a modified administrative alignment MUO; 14 States had pending proposals; 3 States had withdrawn their proposals; and 24 States were not yet participating in the demonstration [23].

The financial alignment or integrated care demonstration projects will be 3 years long and will be evaluated on measures of quality and cost. Participants with full Medicaid and Medicare benefits can participate; although each State can choose to include dual eligible adults over and/or under 65 years old, and will initially limit participation by geographic area. The plans in most States will be implemented by contracts with private managed care insurance companies.

For example, in Ohio, over 100,000 dual eligible beneficiaries are targeted for enrollment in 2014. The program in Ohio will be implemented in seven geographic districts; mostly focused on large urban areas. Ohio initiated a bidding process to allow insurance providers to apply to participate in the demonstration. An MUO requirement is that each region be served by at least two insurance companies. Managed care plans selected to participate in Ohio include: Aetna, Buckeye Community Health, Care Source, Molina Healthcare, and United Community Plan. A controversial aspect of many of the proposals is CMS acceptance of passive enrollment of beneficiaries. Participants would be able to opt out of the Medicare portion of the demonstration; but in most States be required to stay in Medicaid managed care. It is not yet clear what the effects on the demonstrations would be if many of participants decided to opt out of the Medicare portion.

The insurance companies in the capitated model will receive a prospective blended rate that includes payments from CMS for the Medicare portion of covered services and from the State for the Medicaid portion of covered services. CMS is requiring that the agreed upon capitated rate allow for upfront savings for both CMS and the State. CMS is also requiring a quality withhold from the plans' capitated rates; plans could earn back the withheld amount if they meet quality objectives. Although the withhold varies by MUO, it is in the range of 1 % in year 1, 2 % in year 2, and 3 % in year 3 of the demonstrations [24].

The demonstration clinical programs must include full primary care and acute care, mental health, pharmacy, and LTSS benefits. Care coordination is an important component of most of the proposals. This care coordination should include comprehensive care plans for each participant that take into account the patient and families' wishes. The demonstrations will be evaluated on quality measures, including consumer satisfaction, and cost savings. CMS has contracted with the Research Triangle Institute (RTI) to conduct the national evaluation of these demonstrations.

The financial alignment of the demonstrations has created considerable controversy among providers and consumers. For example, nursing home providers are concerned about their future rates and the demonstrations' likely emphasis on home and community-based care. Existing providers of LTSS, such as area agencies on aging, have actively pursued lobbying efforts to ensure that they are included as part of the care management plans of the new managed care plans. Consumer advocacy organizations acknowledge the need for better coordination of services for this vulnerable population, but have been closely monitoring the details of the developing new care systems. Consumer concerns include the proposals for passive enrollment, the size of the clinical networks and disruption of existing care teams, role of consumers in ongoing advisory committees, and restricted home and community based services and transportation (Table 7.2).

Table 7.2 Financial alignment demonstrations – integrating Medicare and Medicaid payment: top consumer concerns

Enrollment in demonstrations should be voluntary via an opt-in process
Delivery systems must have robust provider networks that include a sufficient number of experienced providers
Delivery systems should take steps to allow people to continue seeing long-standing providers
Long-term services and supports (LTSS) needs should be accessed through a comprehensive assessment
An interdisciplinary team should be used to coordinate beneficiaries' care
In addition to the full range of Medicare and Medicaid benefits, states should include additional needed benefits and services, such as, dental, vision, transportation, behavioral diversionary services, etc.
While the demonstration project is being implemented, beneficiaries and advocates should have defined roles at both the state oversight and delivery system levels
Enrollees in demonstrations should be guaranteed a robust set of protections including the freedom to choose their plan, providers, way in which care is delivered, and access to an easy-to-navigate appeals and grievances system
There must be a payment structure that provides sufficient resources to meet the medical and support needs of beneficiaries, especially those with the most complex needs
The state and CMS should rigorously evaluate demonstrations using meaningful and uniform quality measures that evaluate data on beneficiaries' experience, including their level of confidence in taking care of themselves, managing problems, and getting better healthcare and level of involvement in their community
The state and CMS should guarantee dual eligibles a choice of providers who speak their language and understand their culture as well as culturally sensitive written materials

Reprinted with permission from *Generations* 37:2, Summer 2013. Copyright © 2013. American Society on Aging, San Francisco, California. www.asaging.org

Role of Geriatrics and Primary Care Providers in Implementing New Models of Care for the Dual Eligible Beneficiaries

While Fee-For-Service (FFS) Medicare remains the dominant form of health insurance coverage for dual eligibles, pressure to control costs and integrate services is rapidly changing the practice environment for many physicians. The purpose of the new CMS "Duals" office is to help Medicare and Medicaid to work more effectively together. This office is working to speed up the transformation of health services from fragmented, episodic, often duplicative and unnecessary care to comprehensive and integrated services for dual eligibles.

Geriatric Medicine and Primary Care Principles

Geriatric medicine and primary care principles and models of care, if applied to the care of the vulnerable dual eligible population, have the potential to increase quality of care and reduce the cost of services. The ACA initiatives directed at the dual eligible population will more likely be successful if geriatrics and primary care providers participate in planning and direct care provision. Geriatrics providers have the opportunity to display leadership in their communities and institutions to ensure adequate resources to promote patient-centered healthcare outcomes. A few of these principles include:

An important geriatrics strategy is to provide just the *"right" amount of care* (not too much, not too little), in the *"right" location* (usually the least intensive; home is the first choice; the hospital the last choice). To provide the "right" amount of care, the care providers, the patient, and caregivers must develop a care plan that addresses the patient's goals of care. Providing care in the least intensive setting reduces the risk of iatrogenic problems.

Another principle is the importance of *interprofessional teams* in providing care. As the system for providing care to dual eligible beneficiaries is changing, the role of the primary care provider is changing as well. No longer is the physician viewed as the lone provider of health services. Although, the physician is, and will remain, a critical member within the health care team responsible for managing the care of dual eligibles; advance practice registered nurses and physician assistants are playing increasing roles in helping to provide more comprehensive and appropriate health services. The care needs of the dual eligible population are often complex and involves biopsychosocial challenges. Managing patients as a team leads to better continuity, enhanced care coordination, improved patient safety, better chronic illness care, enhanced medication adherence, fewer adverse drug reactions, preserved function, and decreased hospital readmissions [25, 26].

The *Patient-Centered Medical Home (PCMH)* model is not specifically designed for managing dual eligibles or integrating Medicare and Medicaid services. However, this model of high quality primary care is similar to the principles and practices employed by PACE programs which have proven the value of integrated, interprofessional-based care for dual eligible beneficiaries [27]. Health care providers will be valued for their ability to be active, constructive members of a health care team. Working as a member of an interprofessional team, health care providers will need to learn to be effective team players. In the interprofessional environment, such as in PCMH practices, interacting in person or electronically with other health care professionals will be necessary and common. In an interprofessional team setting, face-to-face meetings and discussions with other health professionals to discuss clinical problems and develop plans of care is routine. To be an effective team player, and to engage the assistance of other health professionals, health care providers will need to better understand the role of these other professionals. Knowing what a nurse, social worker, rehabilitation therapist or recreation therapist can and should be able to do, will facilitate primary care providers in their work as team members. It will also allow them to better utilize the resources available to them to the benefit of their patients.

For vulnerable patients living in the community, *enhanced primary care models* have shown promise for improving the care for the vulnerable, functionally impaired patient. For example, the Geriatrics Resources for Assessment and Care of Elders (GRACE) model creates an interprofessional team in the primary care physicians (PCP) office. The team, an advanced practice nurse and social worker, provide home-based geriatrics assessment for vulnerable patients and long-term care management.

The team is supervised by a geriatrician consultant. The care plan is implemented by the entire team under the direction of the PCP. The nurse and social worker coordinate care among all providers and sites of care, utilizing the electronic health record. This model has demonstrated better quality of care for geriatrics syndromes, improvements in health-related quality of life, decreased use of the emergency room, and decreased hospitalizations in high-risk patients [28].

Transitions of care from one setting to another can be dangerous for the vulnerable patient. Poor patient outcomes and frequent hospital readmissions are the result of poorly managed transitions. Evidenced based models to improve care transitions are now available [29, 30]. Key elements that are associated with successful transitional care include:

- Accurate and timely information transfer to the next set of providers.
- Patient and family education about the disease process, self-management recommendations, and expectations at the next level of care.
- Empowerment of patients to assert their preferences for the type, intensity, and location of services.

Emphasizing the quality of visits and procedures rather than volume will become increasingly valued. Under Medicare Fee-For-Service the more providers do, the more providers are paid. This can lead to a misalignment of incentives and poor outcomes. Duplicative or even unnecessary care and services may result. Services that could be provided without a visit may not be performed. Time spent addressing multiple, complex problems that are time consuming are discouraged and avoided. The alignment of financial and quality incentives will promote a more cost effective, evidence-based approach to medicine. With a change in payment structure, spending time to address and resolve complex medical problems, working collaboratively with other team members to avoid institutional care or improve adherence to lifestyle changes, or holding a goals of care discussions with patients and caregivers should be possible.

Electronic Health Records and information technologies will be used to manage disease, prescribe medications, and communicate with other health professionals.

Health providers will need to *know the expectations as well as the policies and practices of the health plans* for which they work. Provider performance will be tracked and measured based on specific processes and procedures. Following appropriate procedures for prescribing medications, using the electronic health record to document clinical care and medications, and adhering to recommended clinical practices are some of the tasks that providers may be expected to perform.

Summary

Geriatrics/gerontology care principles and models of care, if applied to the care of the vulnerable dual eligible population, have the potential to increase quality of care and reduce the cost of services. The ACA initiated demonstrations of the dual eligible population will more likely to be successful if geriatrics providers participate in planning and direct care provision. Geriatrics providers' clinical leadership, when combined with consumer advocacy efforts, is essential to ensure that the financial incentives in the integrated care demonstrations are aligned to ensure optimal care for vulnerable older adults.

References

1. Data book: Beneficiaries dually eligible for Medicare and Medicaid. MedPAC|MACPAC. 2013. http://www.medpac.gov/documents/Dec13_Duals_DataBook.pdf. Accessed 3 June 2014.
2. Henry J Kaiser Family Foundation. Focus on health reform. 2011 (#8192). www.kff.org. Accessed 11 Jan 2013.
3. MEDPAC. Dual eligible beneficiaries. In: A data book: health care spending and the Medicare program. 2011. www.medpac.gov. Accessed 11 Jan 2001.
4. Branch E, Bella M. What is the focus of the integrated care initiatives aimed at Medicare-Medicaid Beneficiaries? J Am Soc Aging. 2013;37:6–12.
5. Davenport K, Hodin RM, Feder J. The "dual eligible" opportunity. Center for American Progress and Community Catalyst. www.americanprogress.org. Accessed 11 Jan 2013.
6. Social Security Act. http://www.ssa.gov/OP_Home/ssact/title18/1812.htm. Accessed 3 June 2014.
7. Frye JE, Center for Medicare Advocacy. Dually eligible for Medicare and Medicaid. Slide presentation at National Health Policy Forum. Washington, DC: Reserve Officers Club; 2003.
8. MEDPAC. Dual eligible beneficiaries: an overview, Chapter 3. In: Report to the congress: new approaches in medicare. Medicare Payment Advisory Commission 2004. pp. 71–92. http://www.medpac.gov/documents/june04_entire_report.pdf. Accessed 18 Jul 2014.
9. Kaiser Family Foundation. Medicaid update: expenditures and beneficiaries in 1994 – policy brief. 1996. http://kff.org/medicaid/issue-brief/medicaid-update-expenditures-and-beneficiaries-in-1994/. Accessed 3 June 2014.
10. Milligan CJ, Woodcock CH. Medicare advantage special needs plans for dual eligibles: a primer. Issue Brief Commonw Fund. 2008;31. 1108
11. Gold M, Jacobson G, Damico A, Neuman T. Issue brief: medicare advantage 2013 spotlight. Kaiser Family Foundation. 2013. http://kaiserfamilyfoundation.files.wordpress.com/2013/06/8448.pdf. Accessed 3 Apr 2014.
12. Medicare Special Needs Plans: A Critical Need for Quality Standards of Care. 2008. http://www.communitycatalyst.org/doc-store/publications/medicare_special_needs_plans_a_report.pdf. Accessed 3 June 2014.
13. Milligan CJ, Woodcock CH. Coordinating care for dual eligibles: options for linking state medicaid programs with medicare advantage special needs plans. Issue Brief Commonw Fund. 2008;1109;32.
14. Medicare Advantage/Part D Contract and Enrollment Data; Special Needs Plans Comprehensive Report. Centers for Medicaid and Medicare Services. 2008. http://www.cms.hhs.gov/MCRAdvPartDEnrolData/. Accessed 4 Apr 2014.
15. PACE in the States. National PACE Association. http://www.npaonline.org/website/download.asp?id=1741&title=PACE_in_the_States. Accessed 4 Apr 2014.
16. Chatterji P, Burstein NR, Kidder D, White A. Evaluation of the Program of All-inclusive Care for the Elderly (PACE) demonstration: the impact of PACE on participant outcomes. Baltimore; Centers for Medicare & Medicaid Services, Department of Health and Human Services. 1998.
17. MEDPAC. Care needs for dual eligibles, Chapter 6. Report to the congress: new approaches in medicare. Medicare Payment Advisory Commission 2004. pp. 145–163. http://www.medpac.gov/documents/june04_entire_report.pdf. Accessed 18 Jul 2014.

18. Burwell B, Saucier P. Managed long-term services and supports programs are a cornerstone for fully integrated care. Generations. 2013;37:33–8.
19. Browdie R. Why is care coordination so difficult to implement? Generations. 2013;37:62–7.
20. Medicare-Medicaid Coordination Office. Centers for Medicare and Medicaid Services. http://www.cms.gov/Medicare-Medicaid-Coordination/Medicare-and-Medicaid-Coordination/Medicare-Medicaid-Coordination-Office/. Accessed 23 Dec 2013.
21. Henry J. Kaiser Family Foundation's. Affordable care act provisions relating to the care of dually eligible Medicare and Medicaid beneficiaries. 2011. http://kff.org/health-reform/issue-brief/affordable-care-act-provisions-relating-to-the/
22. Medicaid Coverage of Medicare Beneficiaries (Dual Eligibles) At a Glance: Medicare Learning Network. Department of Health and Human Services, Centers for Medicare and Medicaid Services. ICN 006977. 2013. http://www.cms.gov/Outreach-and-Education/Medicare-Learning-Network-MLN/MLNProducts/downloads/medicare_beneficiaries_dual_eligibles_at_a_glance.pdf. Accessed 6 Apr 2014.
23. Kaiser Family Foundation. State demonstration proposals to integrate care and align financing and/or administration for dual eligible beneficiaries. 2014. http://kff.org/medicaid/fact-sheet/state-demonstration-proposals-to-integrate-care-and-align-financing-for-dual-eligible-beneficiaries/. Accessed 4 Oct 2014.
24. Kaiser Family Foundation. Explaining the state integrated care and financial alignment demonstrations for dual eligible beneficiaries. 2012. http://kaiserfamilyfoundation.files.wordpress.com/2013/01/8368.pdf. Accessed 23 Dec 2013.
25. Bodenheimer T, Wagner EH, Grumbach K. Improving primary care for patients with chronic illness. JAMA. 2002;288:1775–9.
26. Cohen HJ, Feussner JR, Weinberger M, et al. A controlled trial of inpatient and outpatient geriatric evaluation and management. N Engl J Med. 2002;346:905–12.
27. Hirth V, Baskins J, Dever-Bumba M. Program of All-inclusive Care (PACE): past, present, and future. J Am Med Dir Assoc. 2009;10:155–60.
28. Counsell SR, Callahan CM, Clark DO, Tu W, Buttar AB, Stump TE, et al. Geriatric care management for low-income seniors: a randomized controlled trial. JAMA. 2007;298(22):2623–33.
29. Coleman EA, Parry C, Chalmers S, et al. The care transitions intervention. Arch Intern Med. 2006;166:1822–8.
30. Naylor MD, Aiken LH, Kurtzman ET, et al. The importance of transitional care in achieving health reform. Health Aff. 2011;30:746–54.

Chapter 8
Care Management: From Channeling to Grace

Michael R. Wasserman

It is well known that 79 % of Medicare expenditures are spent on beneficiaries with five or more chronic conditions [1]. This has fueled attempts over the past 40 years to find a better way to manage these patients. When I began my geriatric fellowship in 1988, literature on the Channeling demonstration that tested a case management model in the frail elderly was just being published [2]. I have been fortunate over the past 25 years to have had considerable experience with many case management and care coordination models. It is my hope that by wading through the history of coordinated care programs, and trying to understand not only their purpose, but the outcomes that we seek to achieve through them, that the reader will take a more critical view of programs that attempt to improve quality and lower costs in the care of the Medicare population. I am actually not prepared to accept the notion that even the most robust care coordination model will improve quality or lower costs if performed in isolation to the clinical care of the patient. In fact, it might be possible through an outstanding care coordination program to convince a patient that the world is flat. That would not make it so. On the other hand, chaos is never the best approach to patient care. Overall, the literature has not been kind when it comes to these types of programs. My experience in the healthcare marketplace and examples of successful programs give us reasons for optimism. The GRACE model is an example of a recently successful approach that combines care coordination with expertise in clinical geriatrics [3]. It is my hope that gaining a better understanding of the varying models of care coordination will lead to more clarity regarding effective models of care for a very complex population.

Back in the early 1990s, as a geriatrician with the Southern California Permanente Medical Group, I was a member of a Continuous Quality Improvement (CQI) team that looked at the variation in Medicare hospital utilization rates across various

M.R. Wasserman, M.D. (✉)
Division of Geriatric Medicine, University of Colorado Denver,
22912 Erwin Street, Woodland Hills, CA 91367, USA
e-mail: wassdoc@aol.com

Kaiser facilities. One of the difficult things to prove from a causative perspective was the level of geriatric medical expertise that existed in the facility that had achieved the lowest Medicare hospital utilization rate. Not only did that facility have a geriatric outpatient consultation service, but also had a geriatrician in charge of the hospital discharge planners. We will revisit this issue as we take a further look at the challenges to successful care coordination. Ultimately, our CQI team concluded that one of the key factors that drove higher utilization was the "silo-ing" of care. Different silos within the health care system didn't communicate well with one another, nor were they incentivized to do so. The fact that a health system such as Kaiser-Permanente would identify such issues should give us pause as we go about looking at the history and results of attempts to improve the coordination of care to Medicare beneficiaries.

The fragmented nature of our payment and delivery systems is commonly given as a reason for the high cost of health care in the United States. There are many facets to fragmented care but one of the most prominent is the fact that many Medicare beneficiaries are cared for by multiple specialists. Our existing health care system doesn't assure, nor incentivize, that the care provided by multiple specialists is coordinated. Furthermore, patients receive care and services from home health agencies, physical therapists and a variety of other providers. This care is rarely coordinated or integrated within an entire health care system. Hospitals and private payers will sometimes even provide additional programs to bring patients into their system, but will ultimately not coordinate these programs with the patients primary care physicians or other providers.

The payment system that has evolved under Medicare further exacerbates these critical issues. Paul Starr notes that "in determining physician payment levels, Medicare has for years relied on a private body with no accountability – the subspecialist dominated Relative Value Scale Update Committee of the AMA, now being challenged by primary care physicians because of a pattern of decision making that has contributed to a wide disparity in incomes within the medical profession [4]." Efforts to implement care coordination programs have ultimately run head long into this reimbursement gauntlet. We will discuss efforts to address this later in the chapter.

As a primary care geriatrician for over 25 years, I have had many patients come to me having already been seen by multiple specialists. It has not been uncommon for me to discover that one specialist started a patient on a new medication, and then a side effect from that medication led to a visit to another specialist, and so on and so forth. The most notable example of this occurred a number of years ago in my practice, when I saw a new patient, quite weak and frail, who was on 50 medications! In 1 month, we reduced her medications down to three, and her clinical condition improved dramatically. Lending credence to this concept, Baicker and Chandra found an inverse relationship between specialty care, high costs and quality of care [5]. Patients who identify a specialist as being in control of their care has also been identified as a cause of higher cost of care [6]. Patients themselves even seem to be aware of these issues. In a 2008 survey, 32 % of adults reported experiencing duplicative or unnecessary care [7]. Primary care physicians are also cognizant of the challenges being faced by their own patients. A survey of primary care physicians found that 42 % believed patients in their own practice were receiving too much care [8]. With this as a background, one of the postulates is that the lack of care coordination is an important factor that leads to overtreatment, and that the cost of this in the United States is between $158 and $226 billion annually [9].

There certainly seem to be a lot of people, both physicians and patients alike, who believe that our healthcare system spends too much money. One might pose the question whether the care that is being delivered has been properly conceived, rather than whether it has been well coordinated. Is it possible that the problem actually resides in the hands of clinicians who deliver care that is not evidence-based? It is not clear how coordinating poorly conceived care would improve the quality or lower the costs of care.

The issue of whether Medicare beneficiaries are receiving evidence-based/appropriate care is an important one. The ABIM's "Choosing Wisely" Initiative is a clear indicator of this concern [10]. In a report by the Institute of Medicine, "Crossing the Quality Chasm," geriatric medicine was identified as an area that desperately needs more attention [11]. It has also been noted that training programs for geriatric medicine are underdeveloped [12]. Many of the geriatric residency positions offered remain unfilled. In an article by Schroeder-Mullen, 1998, three reasons were cited for the lack of interest by students to pursue geriatric specialties. The reasons were low reimbursement, the small number of programs offered, and ageist attitudes [12]. In the U.S. most graduates choose the more lucrative specialties avoiding the unpredictable field of geriatrics accompanied by low Medicare reimbursement rates. Furthermore, the effective delivery of care to older adults, and in particular those with multiple chronic illnesses, would benefit from an interdisciplinary team approach to care [13]. Efforts to improve the education and training of clinicians in regards to interdisciplinary teams have shown some promise, but are presently quite limited [14]. These issues increase the challenge of developing coordinated care models for chronically ill individuals.

Looking beyond the purely clinical aspects of fragmented care, in most health care settings there is no single group of participants – physicians, hospitals, public or private payers, or employers – that take full responsibility for guiding the health of a patient or community, so care is distributed across many sites, and integration is lacking or nonexistent [15]. This has led to a variety of attempts over the years to solve the issue of fragmented care, and this effort continues today in the form of the Affordable Care Act (ACA).

The Commonwealth Fund Commission on a High Performance Health System examined the problem of fragmentation in our health care delivery system and also determined it to be a fundamental contributor to poor performance and high costs [16]. They pointed out the following contributing factors (Table 8.1).

Any single one of these factors can have a significant impact on the care of an individual patient. The combination of all four can easily be seen to have an even more dramatic impact on performance and cost. Unfortunately, it could be surmised that solving one of these factors without having an impact on the others will not lead to dramatic improvements. This issue will ultimately be at the crux of any conclusions regarding care coordination as an effective means to improve quality and reduce costs in the care of Medicare beneficiaries.

Table 8.1 Health care delivery system fragmentation

Patients and families navigate unassisted across different providers and care settings, fostering frustrating and dangerous patient experiences
Poor communication and lack of clear accountability for a patient among multiple providers lead to medical errors, waste, and duplication
Absence of peer accountability, quality improvement infrastructure, and clinical information systems foster poor overall quality of care; and
High-cost, intensive medical intervention is rewarded over higher-value primary care, including preventive medicine and the management of chronic illness

Table 8.2 Case management system functions

Identify the full range of services needed
Identify the range of resources available, inclusive of client natural support resources and public community resources
Coordinate the activities of all services and resources
Refer clients to all needed resources
Monitor and follow-up to determine if services are received
Monitor and follow-along to prevent or identify problems in service provision through ongoing contacts with clients, services used, and the clients' natural support resources
Assess and evaluate the effectiveness of all services/resources utilized

It didn't take long after the founding of the Medicare program for there to be some recognition of the issue of fragmented care. In fact, the notion of fragmented care existed long before the founding of Medicare [17], but a program focused on a population with a greater degree of chronic illness was sure to highlight the issue. In this regard, case management and care coordination have long been proposed as a means towards improving the quality of care to the frail elderly, as well as a means towards lowering costs. Caragonne proposed in 1984 a comprehensive approach to case management that focused on service availability, accessibility, responsiveness, continuity, coordination, monitoring/advocacy, and accountability [18]. Case management was felt to be appropriate when clients with multiple problems and needs were unable to define, locate, secure, or retain the necessary resources and services of multiple providers on an ongoing basis. Caragonne proposed that the three key components in case management were accountability, accessibility, and coordination. She proposed a list of the functions in a case management system (Table 8.2).

The inclusion of monitoring, assessment and evaluation of effectiveness certainly was a rational attempt to bring together the various elements that lead to fragmented care. These concepts were not fully understood in the late 1970s, when one of the first models of care coordination, "channeling" was evaluated.

By the late 1970s the potential impact of nursing home placement on the Medicare and Medicaid systems was becoming obvious. Channeling was conceived in order to use comprehensive case management to allocate community services appropriately to the frail elderly in need of long term care. The specific goal of the Channeling program was to enable elderly persons, whenever appropriate, to stay in their own homes rather than entering nursing homes. Channeling financed direct community services, to a lesser or greater degree according to the channeling model, but always as part of a comprehensive plan for care in the community. It had no direct control over medical or nursing home expenditures [2]. In this regard, the Channeling model focused on only one of the key elements that we now know leads to fragmentation of care. Nevertheless, we can learn from the results of the Channeling model.

Channeling was found to increase formal community service use, but did not have a major effect on informal caregiving. Despite success in targeting an extremely frail population, channeling did not substantially reduce nursing home use. The channeling population was frequently hospitalized and made heavy use of physicians and other medical services. The costs of expanding case management and community services were not offset by reductions in nursing home or other costs. The channeling population was also at high risk of dying. Channeling did not affect mortality or measures of client functioning. Channeling reduced unmet needs, increased clients' confidence in receipt of care, and increased their satisfaction with life. Channeling also increased informal caregivers' satisfaction with service arrangements and satisfaction with life.

To summarize, Channeling made patients and caregivers a little happier, but failed to demonstrate any cost savings, which was felt to be due to the lack of impact on clinical care. This has long been the challenge of case management and care coordination models. It should appear obvious that the lack of impact on clinical care would lessen any possibility of having a significant impact on costs, yet attempts to prove otherwise continued to persist in the years following the Channeling study.

One of the more obvious hypotheses for a successful care coordination model is that it must be integrated into the care delivery system in order to work. Enthoven described the concept of an Integrated Delivery System (IDS) as follows: An organized, coordinated and collaborative network that: (1) links various health care providers, via common ownership or contract, across three domains of integration – economic, noneconomic, and clinical – to provide a coordinated, vertical continuum of services to a particular patient population or community and (2) is accountable both clinically and fiscally for the clinical outcomes and health status of the population or community served, and has systems in place to manage and improve them [19].

In endeavoring to implement a successful care coordination program there would thus appear to be four potential models. The first is providing care coordination completely outside of the medical delivery system. The key limiter to this approach is the lack of ability to affect clinical care decisions. There is the additional challenge of achieving cooperation from a patient or caregiver without the approval of their primary care physician or specialist. The literature, which includes the Channeling study, has shown this approach to be problematic. The second approach would be to have outside care coordinators interacting with the patient's physicians. This model has, and continues to be utilized by many health maintenance organizations. On a very practical level, if this method had been shown to be successful in the free market, it would certainly have gained more traction by now. The third approach is to have care coordinators integrated into the primary care provider's practice.

I was fortunate to have had considerable experience with this approach, and I will describe this experience shortly. The fourth approach would be having care coordinators integrated not only into the primary care practice, but into the fabric of the entire health care delivery system. This method fits best into Enthoven's description.

In 1993, GeriMed of America, a geriatric medical management company, was founded by Dr. Jim Riopelle.[1] Dr. Riopelle's background was as an emergency room physician and the first full-time Medical Director for Qual-Med. In both of these capacities, he had seen the impact of fragmented care and attempted to address it through direct intervention, as a medical director, with the patient's physicians. If there was no evidence-based reasoning behind the use of expensive treatment modalities, Dr. Riopelle would speak directly with the patient's physician. By approaching the physician doctor to doctor, he had the ability to discuss any supportive literature or evidence, as well as clinical judgement, that the patient's doctor might have utilized in their decision making process. Such contacts would encourage the physician to give further thought to their clinical decisions, which might result in a change in that decision or in Dr. Riopelle's support, as medical director, for their decision. There were certainly many physicians at the time who saw this approach as intrusive, although it was quite effective. Dr. Riopelle and Qual-Med used this methodology quite successfully in the late 1980s. It is easy to see how this approach would be very dependent on the communication skills of a medical director and would therefore be difficult to translate into a more systemized methodology. In fact, "utilization management", as this was called at the time, has not turned out to be an effective solution to cost containment for Medicare HMO's [20].

Dr. Riopelle ultimately became convinced that delivering care to seniors in a coordinated fashion, led by geriatricians who were trained in the care of older people, would be a cost-effective model of care. At the time, hospitals were able to develop Senior Clinics, utilizing cost-reimbursement in order to cover the overall costs of such a clinic. GeriMed managed such clinics, called MedWise Centers, and each clinic was staffed with geriatricians and a care coordinator [21]. In 1995 a group of geriatricians at GeriMed's first National Medical Directors meeting developed the following "Philosophy of Care" to essentially summarize how geriatricians approach the care of older adults (Table 8.3).

GeriMed's "Philosophy of Care" gives excellent insight into the mindset of geriatricians and summarizes an approach to care that was embedded into their clinical model of care.

Internal GeriMed data at the time demonstrated reduced hospital admissions, shorter hospital length of stays, and lower in-hospital costs. The Balanced Budget Act of 1997 eliminated the cost-reimbursement structure of the hospital based clinics. Not surprisingly, hospitals were not interested in providing their own funding for programs that reduced hospital admission rates in the Medicare population. Without the government's financial support hospitals rapidly fled from this model of care. GeriMed had planned for this eventuality and acquired a few clinics (which it

---

[1] Interview with Dr. Jim Riopelle https://www.twst.com/interview/1408

Table 8.3 GeriMed philosophy of care

Focus on function
Focus on managing chronic disease(s) and developing chronic care treatment models
Identify and manage psychological and social aspects of care
Respect patient's dignity and autonomy
Respect cultural and spiritual beliefs
Be sensitive to the patient's financial condition
Promote wellness
Listen and communicate effectively
Patient centered approach to care, customer focused approach to service
Realistically promote optimism and hope
Team approach to care

quickly expanded) in Central Florida, while assuming full responsibility for a few hospital based clinics in Denver, Colorado. In both markets GeriMed negotiated full risk-contract arrangements with Medicare Advantage plans.

The BBA of 1997 also initiated a 5 year phase-in of risk adjustment for payment to Medicare Advantage plans. Unfortunately, this would prove to come about 5 years too late for GeriMed, whose focus on the frail elderly had already preselected their patient population to be an older, frailer population. This led to losses in the Denver market, which resulted in selling the assets of the clinics and converting a risk-based model to a fee-for-service model, Senior Care of Colorado, PC, in 2001. In Florida, the remaining MedWise Centers continued to be successful, despite the challenges of operating in low AAPCC (Adjusted Average Per Capita Cost) markets, and were ultimately sold when the company was unable to capitalize further expansion.

It is of historical interest that Senior Care of Colorado attempted to maintain a care coordinator model within a fee-for-service environment by offering these services to patients and their families for a fee. This approach was not accepted by patients or caregivers and Senior Care of Colorado was forced to lay off it's care coordinators. Over the next decade, however, Senior Care of Colorado would continue to provide care to thousands of Medicare beneficiaries utilizing a mix of geriatricians, geriatric nurse practitioners and physician assistants. Experience with a local Medicare Advantage plan, once risk-adjustment was factored in, continued to demonstrate cost savings (compared to the rest of the market) from a geriatrician-led primary care model, even without care coordination. This market based successful experience provides significant food for thought in terms of developing successful models of care and can not be ignored.

The underlying reason for the lack of success for GeriMed's clinics in Denver was lack of risk-adjustment. It is an often stated complaint by those who have been unsuccessful in full-risk relationships that "we had a sicker population." It's an easy excuse to make, but fortunately, GeriMed had data to support the fact that the population that they cared for was significantly older and sicker than the typical cohort in the community. Prior to selling the clinics to Senior Care of Colorado, GeriMed prepared an application to be part of Mathematica's Care Coordination Demonstration Project. The patients to be involved in such a project needed to meet certain criteria in order to be deemed of sufficiently high risk. Eighty percent of GeriMed's Denver clinic population met these criteria! All of GeriMed's losses in the market were the result of hospital utilization and Part A costs. With appropriate risk-adjustment, these losses would have been erased and the practice would have been highly profitable. Of note, despite it's high risk population of patient's, GeriMed's Part B costs were still lower than the community norm (not only were there not losses in this area, but there were actual savings), indicating a significantly reduced utilization of specialty care. This reflected the approach to care of a group of geriatricians.

A focus on caring for the most costly Medicare beneficiaries ultimately leads to a discussion of managing chronic illness. In fact, it almost goes without saying that a case management or care coordination program would only be considered in populations with a high degree of chronic illness. While the early literature on this topic didn't put as great a focus on the issue of chronic illness, by the mid 1990s the discussion had clearly turned in that direction. Berenson looked at the issues complicating the management of those with chronic illness across the healthcare landscape. He noted that traditional insurance concepts have significant barriers for delivering care to those with chronic illness (e.g., co-pays decrease the incentive to see a provider) [22]. Arrow had previously commented on the merits of insurance against chronic illness, "on a lifetime insurance basis, insurance against chronic illness makes sense, since this is both highly unpredictable and highly significant in costs. Among people who already have chronic illness, or symptoms which reliably indicate it, insurance in the strict sense is probably pointless [23]." These concerns highlight the great challenges that are faced in trying to implement new models of care in the wake of most health insurance systems, including Medicare.

Berenson also pointed out how the Medicare reimbursement system operates under traditional insurance principles, "nevertheless, despite some loosening of strict insurance principles, a consideration of how Medicare promotes or frustrates improved delivery for patients with chronic conditions must recognize that the traditional Medicare program still functions as an indemnity insurer, and, for the most part, currently is precluded from applying tools used by some private health plans and provider groups to more rationally and effectively manage care for special populations. Reliance of fee for service reimbursement for physician services itself limits delivery system innovation that are available to others [24]." The implementation of care coordination models that are led by primary care physicians have been systematically frustrated by the existing reimbursement decision making process. Part of the problem is that physicians often don't believe that the time they spend in providing care coordination related functions is reimbursable. Furthermore, the reimbursement does not cover the time and work of office staff. Trying to deliver coordinated care in a fee for service practice is therefore seen as having high overhead costs, in a primary care setting already struggling to survive within the existing reimbursement structure.

Berenson attempted to look at other fee-for-service methodologies for the delivery of chronic care. One of the approaches includes the use of telephonic care. He and

Iglehart [25] believed that the cost of billing for telephone care would be high. There are some deficiencies in this viewpoint, insofar as they didn't take into account existing technology (at the time), nor did they consider the option of an hourly rate for care, supported by adequate documentation. Inglehart believed that the audit activities that would have needed to be established to assure proper payments for non-paper communications would be daunting, and certainly more intrusive even than the much criticized oversight requirements for relatively straight forward office visits [26]. This is a somewhat myopic view of the reimbursement system, and certainly should not be a significant factor in determining the value of telephonic management. On the other hand, the fear of an audit will always be an impediment towards the implementation of any new coding system. Berenson also believed that "when phone calls and emails are not reimbursed, conscientious physicians that increase the amount of such contacts will surely suffer financially. In a very real sense, then, the fee for service payment restrictions on reimbursement for non-visit contacts does freeze innovation in how clinical care is practiced [27]."

Ironically, in my experience, many physicians and nurse practitioners will spend time doing work that will be not be reimbursed, in order to do what they perceive is best for the patient. This certainly has reinforced the notion that such types of practices are financially unfeasible. In this regard Berenson was correct, although the providers themselves are often at a loss to understand the full reasons for their financial difficulties. Berenson notes that "a discussion of why prepaid, capitated programs have not achieved better quality outcomes for patients with chronic disease is beyond the scope of this paper [28]." While he doesn't take on the issue of why capitated payments haven't significantly changed models of care and physician behavior, it may be so simple as the fact that if physicians are not trained to care for patients with chronic disease, no degree of incentives will have an impact on that lack of training. If physicians are routinely unable to determine that they are delivering care in a financially unviable manner, it is reasonable to assume that the converse would also be true. If given capitated payments for a particular high risk population, without the proper systems or evidence-based guidelines in place, it would not be surprising that they would not be able to deliver care in a cost-effective manner. This is also what makes both the GeriMed and Senior Care of Colorado work environments interesting. Given the opportunity to practice geriatric medicine in a manner that adhered to GeriMed's "Philosophy of Care," the physicians that worked in this environment felt comfortable with this approach to care. The resulting cost-effective care has been shown to be possible in the marketplace, albeit awaiting substantiation by more rigorous research methods. Nevertheless, one could argue that marketplace success will ultimately trump the need for peer reviewed studies on this topic, if those studies are ever done.

As reimbursement will ultimately be a necessary part of determining an effective model of care, Berenson describes the lengthy process to introduce new codes to support new models of care. "Before speculating on how certain additional services that might help in the management of patients with chronic diseases would be considered, it is important to understand the established procedures CMS has for deciding whether the service will be covered and paid for [29]." This process has historically made the imposition of care coordination models into a medical practice quite difficult. In 2015, 13 years after Berenson wrote about the barriers to new codes, there will finally be CPT codes put in place to pay primary care physicians for the provision of care coordination services within their practice [30]. The history of the use, or lack thereof, of similar codes make the ultimate effectiveness of these new codes questionable. Specifically, the codes for Care Plan Oversight were difficult to implement and were rarely used by primary care practices.

It therefore remains to be seen whether the new codes will be structured in such a way as to facilitate the effective delivery of care coordination within a fee-for-service medical practice. The challenge will be to find ways to integrate the new codes into the practice workflow in a seamless fashion that allows geriatricians and other clinicians with a similar mindset to practice unabated. Furthermore, if the requirements for billing for these services is perceived as increasing the likelihood of an audit, physicians will probably shy away from using these codes.

While attempts to pay for care coordination in the fee-for-service environment continues, there has been some evidence that investments in care coordination in primary care patient centered medical homes does result in reductions in hospital and emergency room utilization [31]. While the overall cost savings have not been shown to be dramatic at this point, this still lends credence to the importance of integrating any care coordination process into the primary care setting.

It is still important to note that most case management demonstrations in the early 1990s did not show any cost savings [32]. One study did demonstrate some impact on overall healthcare costs. It was a randomized controlled study comparing two types of case management for skilled nursing level patients living at home: the centralized individual model and the neighborhood team model [33]. The team model differed from the individual model in that team case managers (which included nurses as well as social workers) performed client assessments, care planning, some direct services, and reassessments; they also had much smaller caseloads and were assigned a specific catchment area. While patients in both groups incurred very high estimated health services costs, the average annual cost during 1983–1985 for team cases was 13.6 % less than that of individual model cases. The lower costs were due primarily to reductions in hospital days and homecare. It should not be surprising that a model that utilized nurses might bring results, again reinforcing the importance of affecting the delivery of clinical care in order to have an impact.

Despite years of negative outcomes for case management programs, The Medicare Coordinated Care Demonstration was authorized by Section 4016 of the Balanced Budget Act of 1997. Mathematica Policy Research subsequently won the award to evaluate and review best practices that came from this demonstration. They identified two main types of coordinated care programs, case management and disease management. Their Best Practices Review pointed out that patients amenable to the two types of interventions differed in important ways. Case management programs served a more select group of frail, disabled patients, at risk for recurrent, costly, recurrent adverse medical events [34]. Disease management programs targeted persons who tended to have a specific condition. Corresponding to the different populations, case management programs tended to individualize care, relying heavily on the judgment of the case manager. In contrast, disease management programs tended to be highly structured and emphasized the use of structured protocols and clinical guidelines.

Fifteen programs were selected from 58 proposals. The programs had to have experience operating a disease management or case management program that had claimed to have reduced hospitalizations or costs in some population or setting. Each program received a negotiated monthly payment for each beneficiary who choose to enroll and was randomized to the treatment group. Payments to the programs ranged from $50 per enrollee per month for low-risk patients with one or more of several chronic illnesses in one program to $437 per month for the first 9 months for all patients with congestive heart failure (CHF) enrolled in another program. The negotiated rates were based on the programs estimates of the cost of their interventions; however, to increase the likelihood that each program would generate net savings to CMS, the rates also were tied to the projected costs of the programs proposed target populations. If a 20 % savings in these projected Medicare costs would not be enough to offset the cost of the intervention, either a program restricted the proposed target population to higher-risk cases (such as beneficiaries with a recent hospitalization) or CMS reduced the proposed program payment to meet this constraint. Five programs had monthly fees exceeding $300; six had fees below $175 [35].

The 15 selected programs varied widely in their organizational structures, target populations, and interventions, and they had varied levels of success in recruiting patients, a consistent issue in trials of this type. The participating organizations included five commercial disease management vendors, three hospitals, three academic medical centers, an integrated delivery system, a hospice, a long-term care facility, and a retirement community. Six programs targeted only a single condition, three served patients with less-specific problems (for example, high-risk patients identified from administrative data by an algorithm), and the six other programs fell between these two extremes [35].

The two programs that lasted the longest in the Demonstration shared some key features. They were case management programs whose target populations included a wide range of chronic conditions. There was a focus in improving patient self-management rather than through the physicians' clinical practice. Care coordinators were highly experienced registered nurses. In-person patient contact was relatively frequent [35].

In 2011, Mathematica Policy Research reported their final findings [36]. Across the board, regardless of the type of program, the results were disappointing. Notably, it was pointed out that none of the 15 programs that participated generated net savings over the original 4-year evaluation period, nine programs definitely increased net costs, three probably increased costs, and three appeared to have been cost neutral and thus were potential candidates for an extension [37].

The demonstration ultimately focused on the two continuing programs, although this was not necessarily a statement as to the success of these programs. They noted that "Care coordination in both programs focused on changing patient behavior rather than physician practice [38]." As we have previously noted, if a model of care does not effect physician practice behavior, it is hard to understand how there can be a

Table 8.4 Mathematica policy research: elements of care to reduce repeat hospitalizations

Face-to-face care coordinator contact with patients
Face-to-face care coordinator contact with physicians
Evidence-based patient education
Management of care setting transitions
Facilitation of communications across providers, and
Medication management

significant impact on either quality or cost of care. Were the outcomes predetermined by the choice of demonstrations? The fact that there were no programs that integrated care coordination into the fabric of the care system and supported a geriatric medical approach to care certainly does not allow us to make any statement in regards to those types of programs and makes it difficult to come to a final conclusion on the topic.

While the results were negative, Mathematica Policy Research determined that several features of the interventions appeared to contribute to the ability to reduce hospitalizations for high-risk patients. Once again we see some of the concepts that we have previously mentioned. They concluded that successful programs were more likely to provide the following six elements of care [39] (Table 8.4).

This brings us to the Affordable Care Act (ACA) and it's attempts to lower costs and improve the quality of care to those with multiple chronic illnesses. Section 3022 of the ACA established the Medicare Shared Savings Program for accountable care organizations (ACOs) as a potential solution to fragmentation and the high costs of health care. The creation of ACOs was one of the first delivery reform initiatives that were implemented under the ACA. Under the law, an ACO assumed responsibility for the care of a clearly defined population of Medicare beneficiaries attributed to it on the basis of their patterns of use of primary care. Berwick, while describing the Medicare Shared Savings Program for Accountable Care Organizations, stated, like many before him, that "fragmentation leads to waste and duplication – and unnecessarily high costs [15]." He and others clearly believe that the ACA provides for programs that will reduce fragmentation. If an ACO then succeeds in both delivering high-quality care and reducing the cost of that care to a level below what would otherwise have been expected, it will share in the Medicare savings it achieves [15].

ACOs, as established by the ACA, are certainly not the first attempt by the government to address the issue of fragmentation through new legislated programs. During the 1980s and 1990s, the concept of managed care, through health maintenance organizations (HMOs), were supposed to address this and other issues. While some have deemed managed care to have been a failure [40], similar models continue to dominate attempts to reduce costs in an ever more expensive health care environment. In many ways, conceptually, an ACO is just another format for managed care concepts. Some have tried to argue that ACOs are different than their HMO counterparts but their arguments tend to focus around the availability of newer technology and the fact that patients don't actually sign up to be part of an ACO [41]. What is clear is that the theory that an ACO will lower the costs of care is predicated on coordination and integration of care as well as financial incentives.

In the 1990s Disease Management Programs were also promoted as the solution to the increasing costs of Medicare. Oxford Health, Humana, and others either implemented their own programs or outsourced Disease Management Programs. Oxford Health was quite proud of their programs, promulgating the notion that each of these programs was saving lots of money. Then, in October of 1997, despite a multitude of "successful" Disease Management Programs, Oxford Health declared significant losses in their Medicare program and their stock dropped precipitously [42]. As was previously noted, the Medicare Coordinated Care Demonstration included five Disease Management Programs. Without a focus on changing physician behavior towards a more geriatric friendly approach, it should now be easy to see how these programs were all doomed to failure. Will there be any difference in ACO's or other programs supported by the ACA? It is hard to see how there will be. Incentives alone clearly do not lead to successful care management programs. Ultimately, a successful program must change physician's practice behavior.

This chapter opened with the statement that 79 % of Medicare expenditures are spent on patients with multiple chronic conditions. In keeping with a focus on this issue, Wagner developed a Chronic Care Model (CCM) that was based on a group of concepts meant to functionally address chronic disease management [43]. It was "designed to help practices improve patient health outcomes by changing the routine delivery of ambulatory care through six interrelated system changes meant to make patient-centered, evidence-based care easier to accomplish. The aim of the CCM was to transform the daily care for patients with chronic illnesses from acute and reactive to proactive, planned, and population-based. It was designed to accomplish these goals through a combination of effective team care and planned interactions; self-management support bolstered by more effective use of community resources; integrated decision support; and patient registries and other supportive information technology (IT). These elements were designed to work together to strengthen the provider-patient relationship and improve health outcomes [44]." Nolte and McKee, in evaluating the success of the CCM concluded, "In summary, as judged by the published literature, the evidence remains inconclusive on the impact of applying the CCM as a whole on quality of care and patient outcomes, as does the evidence about which components, in what combination, achieve the greatest improvements of what process, output and/or outcome measures [45]." On the other hand, Wagner's model might work brilliantly if it was put in place with actual evidence-based literature for Medicare beneficiaries with multiple chronic conditions. Unfortunately, this literature is presently lacking. Once again, geriatricians with considerable clinical experience might be expected to practice in a fashion that would reflect this approach to care. Furthermore, geriatricians are typically trained to operate within an interdisciplinary team, and having a team whose members are also trained in geriatrics (e.g., geriatric nurse specialist, geriatric pharmacist, etc.) could prove particularly valuable.

Even if we had the clinicians to deliver the care, whether any of these models can work is still constrained by the ability to implement them, if not in the primary care providers office, then in any health care system. How to pay for a model, even if it is deemed to be effective, will still impact the ability to implement the model. Essential

Hospitals Institute, in their Integrated Health Care Literature Review notes that, "to reduce costs, physicians and hospitals require a payment system that is based on value (quality and cost) rather than volume, most likely in the form of advanced payment. But advanced payment methods are most feasible in highly organized, integrated systems of care. Without payment reform, physicians and hospitals have little incentive to integrate. But without integrated systems, advanced payment systems are difficult to test and implement [46]." Hence, we have a conundrum.

In order to impact the care of high risk older adults, it is clear that case management models that don't directly influence the medical care of the individual do not work. We will now discuss a few models that have demonstrated success in order to hone in on the factors that can be attributed to positive outcomes. We have already noted the paucity of geriatricians and other clinicians trained in geriatrics. The lack of training in certain core competencies in geriatrics might be considered to be at the heart of the problem of providing coordinated care to high risk patients. Finding a way to actually evaluate and influence medical decisions in a manner consistent with core geriatric principles was the basis for the development of the GRACE model [3]. The GRACE intervention includes an advanced practice nurse and social worker (GRACE support team) who care for seniors in collaboration with the patient's primary care physician and a geriatrics interdisciplinary team led by a geriatrician. In the clinical trial evaluating the effectiveness of this model, the GRACE support teams were employed by the primary care practice. They met with the patient in the home to conduct an initial comprehensive geriatric assessment and then presented their findings to the larger GRACE interdisciplinary team during the next weekly meeting to develop an individualized care plan, which included activation of GRACE protocols and corresponding team suggestions for evaluating and managing common geriatric conditions. The team then met face-to-face with the patient's primary care physician to discuss and modify the plan. Collaborating with the physician and supported by the GRACE interdisciplinary team, the support team then implemented the plan consistent with the patient's goals through face-to-face and telephone contacts with patients, family members or caregivers, and health care professionals. Each patient received a minimum of one in-home follow-up visit to review the care plan, one telephone or face-to-face contact per month, and a face-to-face home visit after any emergency department (ED) visit or hospitalization. Otherwise, the number, timing, and content of additional patient contacts occurred as appropriate to implement the care plan. An annual in-home reassessment starts the process over again [3].

The GRACE intervention demonstrated a reduction in hospital days and ER visits in the high risk group [3]. Costs of the GRACE intervention in the high risk group after 2 years trended lower but statistically was reported to be cost neutral [47]. There is now data available that found a statistically significant reduction in costs over 3 years. Based on the powering of a study such as this with an "n" of about 200 patients, it is not surprising that an intervention such as this might take 3 years in order to demonstrate statistically significant cost reductions. Ironically, in my experience most actuaries require 5,000 Medicare lives in order to avoid the risk of significant outliers.

Table 8.5 Grace intervention

NP/SW team assigned by physician and practice site
Focus on geriatric conditions and medication management to complement primary care
Provided recommendations for care and resources for implementation and follow-up
Incorporated proven care transition strategies
Provided home-based and proactive care management
Integrated with community resources and social services, and
Developed relationships through longitudinal care

With this in mind, the GRACE intervention has also been implemented in a large managed care medical group in Southern California. The targeted population were 174 homebound patients. This was not a randomized controlled trial, and there is always the probability of regression towards the mean, but the intervention found the following reductions in utilization: 34 % decrease in hospital admissions, 29 % decrease in hospital bed days, 44 % decrease in sub acute admits, 53 % decrease in sub-acute bed days, and 22 % decrease in ED visits [48].

The key elements that were felt to be important for the success of the GRACE model [49] are listed in (Table 8.5).

So, as we approach the full implementation of the ACA, where does all of this information leave us? Since Medicare is a federally legislated program, we really should look no further than CMS to determine the state of mind at CMS as it relates to the testing and implementation of new programs. Jonathon Blum, Director, Center for Medicare Management on Improving Quality, in a statement to congress in 2011, stated that "CMS has established initiatives to ensure that Medicare patients get the right care, in the right place, at the right time. A key part of CMS' work in this area is a multi-part initiative built around Accountable Care Organizations (ACOs), which bring together doctors, hospitals and other health care providers to better coordinate care for patients. ACOs are an innovative service delivery model being used by CMS and in the private sector and communities across the country. If ACOs improve quality of care and lower costs, health care providers, as well as Medicare, can share in the savings. Those savings will help to shift payment incentives toward rewarding quality and value rather than volume of care. Provider participation in ACOs is purely voluntary, and beneficiaries will continue to have all their same benefits, including their ability to see any Medicare provider."[2]

Blum also pointed out that CMS is using its new authorities through the Center for Medicare and Medicaid Innovation (the Innovation Center) to test alternative payment models and prepare organizations to provide accountable care.

---

[2] Statement by Jonathan Blum, Director, Center for Medicare Management on Improving Quality, Lowering Costs: The Role of Health Care Delivery System before Committee on Homeland Health, Education, Labor and Pensions. United States Senate Thursday November 10, 2011.

These initiatives include: "The Pioneer ACO Model, which is designed for health care organizations and providers with experience in coordinating care for patients across settings,"[3] "The Advance Payment ACO Model, which will provide additional support to rural and physician-based ACOs who want to participate in the Medicare Shared Savings Program, but lack the start-up resources to build the necessary infrastructure, such as new staff or information technology systems. The advance payments would be recovered from any future shared savings which ACO earns through performance,"[4] and, "The Accelerated Development Learning Sessions, which are available for providers interested in learning more about the steps necessary to become an ACO."[5]

Blum has clearly bought into the idea that ACO's will be an important solution to the problem of fragmentation and high costs in the Medicare program. Unfortunately, while an ACO might reduce fragmentation, there really is little evidence that it will lower costs. The exception to this would be an ACO that integrates a geriatric medical care approach into the fabric of its delivery model. I will leave a further discussion of ACO's and their ability to impact the cost and quality of care to other authors in this text.

In the aftermath of the passing and ongoing implementation of the Affordable Care Act, the concept of High Value Primary Care [50] has also been gaining traction in congress. This appears to be the latest attempt to harness an out of control health care system. Not surprisingly, the concept is intertwined with the integration of care coordination and case management services within the primary care setting as part of the Comprehensive Primary Care Initiative [51]. This initiative provides funding to allow for care management services in primary care practices, but does not assure the necessary training to prepare an appropriately trained workforce to care for high risk patients with multiple chronic diseases. So, while this is a step forward in terms of providing integrated care coordination, it is still lacking insofar as it doesn't assure a care delivery system based on geriatric medical principles. We will have to await the results of this effort.

The GeriMed MedWise Center model and the Senior Care of Colorado models were never validated in a rigorous research environment. However, they both achieved financial success in the marketplace. The GRACE model takes a similar approach to influencing the care of patients in the primary care setting. At the present time, there is one pertinent model that has been studied and tested extensively. It is perhaps the most studied model of fully integrated care coordination within a geriatric focused care model. It is the Program of All-Inclusive Care of the Elderly (PACE) program [52, 53].

PACE is a comprehensive community-based care model for frail, chronically ill older adults whose significant functional and cognitive impairments make them

---

[3] Ibid.
[4] Ibid.
[5] Ibid.

nursing home eligible. The first program, On Lok, initially offered adult day care with comprehensive medical services, rehabilitation services, respite, and social services. The cost of care for the participants in the original program was 15 % less than traditional fee-for-service care. It is both ironic and telling that in the early 1980s this finding did not lead to any further evaluation of the program in an outpatient setting. PACE was focused on keeping nursing home eligible seniors, a very high risk population, in the community. PACE offers all Medicare and Medicaid services through a single point of delivery targeted to frail elderly with a host of chronic care needs. It is a provider-based model of care, with participants at the center of the plan of care developed by an interdisciplinary team of health care providers. The model offers access to the full continuum of preventive, primary, acute, rehabilitative, and long-term care services. PACE programs take many familiar elements of the traditional health care system and reorganize them in a way that provides comprehensive care in a fiscally responsible manner for families, health care providers, government programs, and others that pay for care [54]. PACE programs have historically been staffed by geriatricians, which is not surprising insofar as the focus is based on geriatric medical principles.

PACE programs have been shown to improve the quality of care and access to services based on need. Significant outcomes across all PACE programs include greater adult day health care use, lower skilled home health visits, fewer hospitalizations, fewer nursing home admissions, higher contact with primary care, longer survival rates, an increased number of days in the community, better health, better quality of life, greater satisfaction with overall care arrangements, and better functional status [55]. The PACE program is an expensive program that focuses on the highest cost Medicare beneficiaries. It has been successful. Translating this program upstream to slightly less vulnerable individuals would require lower costs than the PACE program presently spends in order to provide it's approach to care. While this is a challenge, it is probably where the focus needs to lie as we attempt to develop a truly effective integrated care coordination model with a geriatric medical focus at its core.

Based on the existing literature it appears that care coordination in and of itself is not sufficient as a means to improve quality and reduce costs. If costly, non-evidence based treatments are the clinical norm in a community, then no amount of care coordination will significantly improve quality outcomes or cost. On the other hand, if care coordination provides a means to disseminate evidence-based information so as to impact the actual delivery of care, and by coordinating that care assures that it is delivered in the most effective manner possible, then the results have the potential to follow. This method does open the door to the potential for outcomes based reimbursement, albeit the definitive outcomes in the frail older adult population do not exist at this time. Nevertheless, the literature from successful programs and my experience in the marketplace would suggest that clinicians well trained in geriatric medicine, operating in an environment where core competencies in geriatrics are assured, and that supports coordinated care utilizing the concepts outlined in this chapter, have the best opportunity to improve quality and lower costs in the care of Medicare beneficiaries.

References

1. Anderson G. Chronic care: making the case for ongoing care. Princeton: The Robert Wood Johnson Foundation; 2010. p. 18.
2. Kemper P, Mathematica Policy Research, Inc., et al. The evaluation of the national long term care demonstration: final report executive summary. Washington, DC: U.S. Department of Health & Human Services; 1986.
3. Counsell SR, Callahan CM, Clark DO, et al. Geriatric care management for low-income seniors: a randomized controlled trial. JAMA. 2007;298:2623–33.
4. Starr P. The Medicare bind. American Prospect (November 2011), p. 32.
5. Baicker K, Chandra A. Medicare spending, the physician workforce, and beneficiaries' quality of care. Health Aff. 2004. doi:10.1377/hlthaff.w4.18.
6. Reschovsky JD, Hadley J, Saiontz-Martinez CB, Boukus ER. Following the money: factors associated with the cost of treating high-cost medicare beneficiaries. Health Serv Res. 2011;46(4):997–1021.
7. How S, et al. Public views on U.S. Health System Organization: a call for new directions. New York: Commonwealth Fund; 2008.
8. Sirovich B, et al. Too little? Too much? Primary care physicians' views on US health care: a brief report. Arch Intern Med. 2011;171(17):1582–5.
9. Berwick D, Hackbarth A. Eliminating waste in U.S. health care. J Am Med Assoc. 2012;307(14):1513–6.
10. Cassel CK, Guest JA. Choosing wisely, helping physicians and patients make smart decisions about their care. JAMA. 2012;307(17):1801–2.
11. Institute of Medicine. Crossing the quality chasm: a new health system for the 21st century. Washington, DC: National Academy Press; 2001.
12. Schroeder-Mullen H. Reframing the geriatric patient. JAMA. 1998;279(13):1034.
13. Partnership for Health in Aging. Position statement on interdisciplinary team training in geriatrics: an essential component of quality healthcare for older adults. March, 2011, http://www.americangeri-atrics.org/files/documents/pha/PHA_Full_IDT_Statement.pdf.
14. Dyer CB, Hyer K, Feldt KS, et al. Frail older patient care by interdisciplinary teams: a primer for generalists. Gerontol Geriatr Educ. 2003;24(2):51–62.
15. Berwick DM. Launching accountable care organizations – the proposed rule for the medicare shared savings program. N Engl J Med. 2011;364:e32. doi:10.1056/NEJMp1103602.
16. Shih A, Davis K, Schoenbaum SC, et al. Organizing the U.S. health care delivery system for high performance. New York: The Commonwealth Fund; 2008.
17. Starr P. The social transformation of American medicine, New York: Basic Books, 1982, p. 196.
18. Hubbard Linz M, McAnally P, Wieck C, editors. History of case management: historical, current, and future perspectives. Papers presented at a conference co-sponsored by the Minnesota University Affiliated Program on Developmental Disabilities and the Minnesota Department of Human Service, Minneapolis, 1986.
19. Enthoven AC. Integrated delivery systems: the cure for fragmentation. Am J Manag Care. 2009;15:S284–90.
20. Hurley RE, Bannick RR. Utilization managers in Medicare risk contract HMOs: from control to collaboration. QRB Qual Rev Bull. 1993;19(4):131–7.
21. Wasserman MR, Holthaus KM, Cosgrove K. TheMedWiseCenter–an innovation in primary care geriatrics. Continuum. 1998;18(1):18–23.
22. Berenson RA. Confronting the barriers to chronic care management in medicare. Prepared for the study panel on Medicare and chronic care in the 21st century, Washington, D.C: National Academy of Social Insurance April 2002, p. 3
23. Arrow KJ. Uncertainty and the welfare economics of medical care. Am Econ Rev. 1963;LIII(5):941–73.

24. Berenson RA. Confronting the barriers to chronic care management in Medicare. Prepared for the study panel on Medicare and chronic care in the 21st century, National Academy of Social Insurance, Washington, D.C. April 2002, p. 5–6.
25. Iglehart JK. The centers for medicare and medicaid services. N Engl J Med. 2001;345(26): 1920–4.
26. Berenson RA. Confronting the barriers to chronic care management in Medicare. Prepared for the study panel on Medicare and chronic care in the 21st century, National Academy of Social Insurance, April 2002, p. 6.
27. Berenson RA. Confronting the barriers to chronic care management in Medicare. Prepared for the study panel on Medicare and chronic care in the 21st century, National Academy of Social Insurance, April 2002, p. 7.
28. Berenson RA. Confronting the barriers to chronic care management in Medicare. Prepared for the study panel on Medicare and chronic care in the 21st century, National Academy of Social Insurance, April 2002, p. 14.
29. Berenson RA. Confronting the barriers to chronic care management in Medicare. Prepared for the study panel on Medicare and chronic care in the 21st century, National Academy of Social Insurance, April 2002, p. 24.
30. Schneider ME. Medicare finalizes plan to pay PCPs for care beyond the office visit. Intern Med News. 2013;46(20):1.
31. Grumbach K, Grundy P. Outcomes of implementing patient centered medical home interventions: a review of the evidence from prospective evaluation studies in the United States. Washington, DC: Patient-Centered Primary Care Collaborative; 2010.
32. Schore JL, Brown RS, Cheh VA. Case management for high cost Medicare beneficiaries. Health Care Financ Rev. 1999;20:87–101.
33. Eggert GM, Zimmer JG, Hall WJ, Friedman B. Case management: a randomized controlled study comparing a neighborhood team and a centralized individual model. Health Serv Res. 1991;26(4):471–507.
34. Eggert GM, Zimmer JG, Hall WJ, Friedman B. Case management: a randomized controlled study comparing a neighborhood team and a centralized individual model. Health Serv Res. 1991;26(4):32.
35. Brown R, Peikes D, Chen A, et al. The evaluation of the Medicare coordinated care demonstration: findings for the first two years. Princeton: Mathematica Policy Research; 2007.
36. Schore J, et al. Fourth report to congress on the evaluation Mathematica Policy Research of the Medicare coordinated care demonstration, March 2011.
37. Schore J, et al. Fourth report to congress on the evaluation Mathematica Policy Research of the Medicare coordinated care demonstration, March 2011, p. 2.
38. Schore J, et al. Fourth report to congress on the evaluation Mathematica Policy Research of the Medicare coordinated care demonstration, March 2011, p. 6.
39. Schore J, et al. Fourth report to congress on the evaluation Mathematica Policy Research of the Medicare coordinated care demonstration, March 2011, p. 16.
40. Robinson JC. The end of managed care. JAMA. 2001;285(20):2622–8.
41. Emanuel EJ. Why accountable care organizations are not 1990s managed care redux. JAMA. 2012;307(21):2263–4. doi:10.1001/jama.2012.4313.
42. CNN Money. Oxford infection spreads. http://money.cnn.com/1997/10/27/companies/oxford/. Accessed 27 Oct 1997.
43. Wagner E. Chronic disease management: what will it take to improve care for chronic illness? Eff Clin Pract. 1998;1:2–4.
44. Coleman K, Austin BT, Brach C, Wagner EH. Evidence on the chronic care model in the new millennium. Health Aff. 2009;28(1):75–85. doi:10.1377/hlthaff.28.1.75.
45. Nolte E, McKee M. Caring for people with chronic conditions: a health system perspective, Chapter 4. Maidenhead: Open University Press/McGraw-Hill, 2008, 64–91.
46. Integrated Health Care Literature Review. Washington, DC: America's Essential Hospitals; May 2013, p. 1.
47. Counsell SR, Callahan CM, Tu W, et al. Cost analysis of the geriatric resources for assessment and care of elders care management intervention. JAGS. 2009;57:1420–6.

48. Counsell SR, Frank K, Levine S, et al. Dissemination of GRACE care management in managed care medical group. AGS Poster, May 2011.
49. Counsell SR. GRACE Team Care. SNP Alliance, October 2013.
50. Baron RJ, Davis K. Accelerating the adoption of high-value primary care – a new provider type under Medicare? N Engl J Med. 2014;370(2):99–101.
51. From the Centers for Medicare and Medicaid Services. http://innovation.cms.gov/Files/x/CPC_PracticeSolicitation.pdf.
52. Boult C, Wieland GD. Comprehensive primary care for older patients with multiple chronic conditions: "nobody rushes you through". JAMA. 2010;304(17):1936–43.
53. Hirth V, Baskins J, Dever-Bumba M. Program of all-inclusive care (PACE): past, present, and future. J Am Med Dir Assoc. 2009;10:155–60.
54. Hirth V, Baskins J, Dever-Bumba M. Program of all-inclusive care (PACE): past, present, and future. J Am Med Dir Assoc. 2009;10:157.
55. Hirth V, Baskins J, Dever-Bumba M. Program of all-inclusive care (PACE): past, present, and future. J Am Med Dir Assoc. 2009;10:158.

Chapter 9
Program Evaluation: Defining and Measuring Appropriate Outcomes

Peter A. Hollmann

The major legislation to expand healthcare insurance coverage has failed. Health care expenditures are not sustainable. They are the fastest growing part of the federal budget and threaten the stability of our national economy. Household economies are also threatened with bankruptcy due to medical costs. Our volume based payment system results in a built hospital bed being a filled hospital bed and many unnecessary procedures. Conversely, there are rampant gaps in care with the standards of care being met only half of the time. Medical errors kill thousands. Our educational and training system does not produce the workforce we need. Our technology enamored country diffuses unproven technology as professionals and institutions engage in arms races over the newest devices. As healthcare consumes a growing portion of the gross domestic product, it limits our ability to spend on other worthy areas such as better housing, infrastructure and education – which may actually contribute more to population health than healthcare does. As the cost of health insurance becomes a greater proportion of employee costs, even potentially eclipsing wages, employees are afraid to change jobs, employers drop coverage and America's products become non-competitive in global markets. Our manufacturing base declines, the middle class erodes and there is economic polarization as the American dream slips away from too many. Without a doubt, the landmark legislation signed into law by our President is a failure.

The president is Lyndon Baines Johnson. The year is 1965 and the law is Medicare.

Most of the healthcare professionals, economists and experts of that day have gone on to become Medicare beneficiaries and died. The debate of that era over Medicare was not that different from today's debate over the Affordable Care Act (ACA). Who today really believes Medicare is a failure? If the belief is that it is a

---

P.A. Hollmann, M.D. (✉)
Division of Geriatrics, Blue Cross & Blue Shield of Rhode Island,
500 Exchange Street, Providence, RI 02903-2699, USA
e-mail: Peter.Hollmann@bcbsri.org

success, even if a flawed success, what measures define success or failure? The problems outlined above all exist today, even if some would choose to debate fine points. Undeniably, Medicare has played a major role in shaping the healthcare system and country that we have today. The access to healthcare for seniors and those with conditions such as End Stage Renal Disease would be markedly diminished without Medicare. Healthcare today is much more effective than in 1965 and has played a role in extending the average life expectancy. The addition of Medicaid greatly enhanced access to care for children and those with disabilities and those needing long-term care. In thinking about whether Medicare has been a success or failure or both, we can conceptualize its evaluation because it is a familiar subject. It helps us understand the process and challenges of evaluating the ACA. It also reminds us that regardless of technical accuracy, scholarly research and statistical prowess, in the end public opinion may be the only evaluation that truly matters.

The ACA addresses health insurance, healthcare quality and payment methods designed to promote quality. It builds upon activities already in progress at state and/or federal levels. The goal is to achieve the "Triple Aim" and, in doing so, create a stronger and better America in ways that go beyond health. The Triple Aim has been phrased in slightly different ways at different times and by different users, but is:

- Improving the patient experience of care (including quality and satisfaction);
- Improving the health of populations; and
- Reducing the per capita cost of health care.

What measures will be appropriate to define success in this goal is a complex question. The purpose of this chapter is to explore measures, measurement and use of measurement. The focus is on healthcare quality, but the measures of quality derive from greater goals related to health and economics. Ultimately, it is the intended or eventual use of measurement that matters most. It is the use that will both drive improvement and drive debate. Current measures and measurement are inadequate to the task of providing definitive answers to most meaningful questions ranging from the efficacy of a massive piece of legislation such as the ACA or the quality of care provided by an individual clinician. The process of seeking how best to quantify and promote success will, in itself, be an exercise in quality improvement that must be undertaken if we are to advance our goal of achieving the Triple Aim. The approach used in this chapter is one that is designed to create an overview for clinicians. It is not written for the expert analyst or statistics authority, who will likely recognize some liberties taken for the sake of providing general information.

The Affordable Care Act

The ACA might be boiled down into having two basic goals: increase access to health care by changing health insurance and improve the value of healthcare. Health is a critical attribute of happiness and wellbeing. It is also a critical attribute of a productive society. Health is affected by genetics, habits/lifestyle, medical care, the environment, wealth, education and many interacting factors. Accordingly, in the vision of Barack Obama, the impact of the ACA is to extend well beyond health, health insurance and quality of care. The President's words of March 5, 2009, place the ambition of the ACA – and therefore, one could argue, the standards by which its success is to be measured – in an expansive social and economic context:

> At the fiscal summit that we held here last week, the one thing on which everyone agreed was that the greatest threat to America's fiscal health is not Social Security, though that's a significant challenge; it's not the investments that we've made to rescue our economy during this crisis. By a wide margin, the biggest threat to our nation's balance sheet is the skyrocketing cost of health care. It's not even close.

Consider the breadth of metrics that could be used to define the success of the ACA in light of this broad vision. Not only will the health of populations be used to define quality and efficiency of care by providers and the payment the providers receive, the health of the population will define the successes and failures of the ACA itself. Here are some provisions of the law followed by some potential or current measures by which the success of those provisions might be assessed:

Increase the number of individuals with health insurance by providing access to coverage, financial support and a personal mandate for coverage: the percent of the population with insurance coverage that includes essential benefits; the percent of those at specific income levels with coverage; the percent of younger individuals who purchase coverage through an exchange; the number of businesses that increase or drop employer sponsored coverage; percent of family income going to healthcare; the rate of medical cost driven personal bankruptcy.

Expand eligibility for Medicaid through federal support of state initiatives: The number of newly insured; the number of conversions of private coverage to Medicaid; the financial stability of providers as Medicaid expands; the number of providers accepting Medicaid; state budget surplus or deficit.

Create a competitive marketplace with specific ground rules such as essential benefits, ending lifetime or annual caps and pre-existing condition exclusions and using risk adjusted payments to health plans: market choice; premium stability over time; customer satisfaction and plan stability in enrollments; less "cherry picking" (i.e., tactics to avoid adverse selection such as excluding providers with complex patients from the network).

Improve value by paying for quality or penalizing undesirable outcomes, such as the Medicare Advantage 5 Star Program or Hospital Acquired Conditions penalties: improvements in the quality measures that are used in these programs; improvements in quality measures that are not used in payment; market share of higher performing organizations; beneficiary choice; stability of safety net organizations; reduction in the growth of the rate of the portion of the gross domestic product (GDP) and federal budget spent on health care.

Require first dollar coverage for preventive services: the percent of the population that receives the recommended service; reductions in the target illness morbidity and mortality; reductions in the cost of care for the targeted conditions; fewer days of disability or missed work; increased average life expectancy; increased average life expectancy and decreased disability for lower socio-economic status populations; fewer unintended pregnancies.

Promote rapid diffusion of cost effective care and system redesign through the creation of programs related to comparative effectiveness and innovation: lower total cost of care trends; optimal care is better defined and new measures of care are defined; population health status improves; hospital readmissions are reduced.

Each listed measure could also be joined by broader measures that reflect the social context of healthcare. For example, better physical and mental health could improve employee productivity and the growth of the GDP. Less money spent on healthcare and fewer medical bankruptcies could mean that affordable housing receives greater attention, more people have rent money and homelessness decreases. Innovative care models may even use healthcare funds for transportation or housing, if that is what it takes to manage the health care costs of certain individuals, further reducing homelessness. Fewer unintended pregnancies may reduce the crime rate.

Principles of Quality Measurement

The almost limitless expansion of evaluation and measurement of the ACA provided above may seem foolish. But it makes a point about keeping an end goal in mind. Diabetes is a condition familiar to most everyone and certainly all healthcare professionals. We measure whether hemoglobin A1c is performed. Do we care if a hemoglobin A1c is performed? No, we really care about the result being optimized. We measure whether the hemoglobin A1c is within a target range. Do we care about the hemoglobin A1c result? No, we really care about avoiding end organ complications of diabetes such a stroke, heart attack, amputation, blindness and kidney failure. Do we care about end organ complications in people with advanced dementia who have diabetes? Probably not, but we care about their comfort. Is there evidence that measuring and controlling the hemoglobin A1c in a person with advanced dementia improves comfort? It is unlikely there is. The converse is just as probable. We care about access to affordable health insurance because lack of health insurance is associated with death, disability and lost productivity, not because we really care about insurance.

Measurement of quality and the outcomes of healthcare is an exercise in compromise: guidelines do not apply to every patient; only major exceptions can be included in measures; data collection must be efficient and therefore may rely upon information primarily submitted for payment purposes; and risk adjustment is impossible or imperfect. For this reason, the intended use of the measure is critical. The intended use should define the selection criteria and measurement methodology. For example, an internally defined measure may be just what is needed to assess the impact of a rapid cycle quality improvement process. However, such a measure would be inappropriate to compare two providers in different regions. Some measures may effectively be used in comparing certain provider types, but not others. For example, a surgical infection rate is much more likely to be related to the facility and its team of providers than an individual surgeon. It is generally true that the broad intent of measurement is to improve health by improving healthcare.

It is impossible to assess interventions unless there is measurement, and the adage is that one cannot improve what one cannot measure.

In order to better understand quality measures in health care an overview may be useful. In the 1960s Avis Donabedian described a model of defining quality that looked at three attributes: **structure, process and outcomes**. This model remains relevant. The definition of "outcomes" may vary depending on whether the use is a clearly relevant patient oriented outcome such as death or whether it is an intermediate, proxy or short term "outcome" such as an LDL level that is truly not an outcome at all, but is a result of a process of care. Each type of these measures or attributes of quality have a role in evaluation and improvement. However, for any of them to be meaningful, the measure must ultimately be linked to an outcome that is meaningful such as death, function or comfort.

An example of a structural measure would be whether a Medicare Accountable Care Organization (ACO) has a governance structure that requires organizational leadership from a person with competencies in geriatric care. This may make sense from a theoretical point of view, but ideally it is bolstered by evidence that such a structure leads to better results clinically or in cost or both. Structural measures are often "standards" and tend to be readily defined and measured. Nursing hours per patient is a structural measure that Medicare has adopted for nursing facility performance measurement (Medicare.gov Nursing Home Compare).

Process measures are those that evaluate the process of care. Whether an appropriate perioperative antibiotic was given at the right time or not for a specified surgical procedure is a process measure used in Medicare (Medicare.gov Hospital Compare). These types of measures are widely used. A major advantage of process measures is that they require much less risk adjustment in use than an outcome measure. If everything in control of the health care team was done properly and the patient died anyway, then it must have been due to uncontrollable factors and the care was good despite the outcome, or so it is theorized. Even process measures may require consideration of the types of factors that might be labelled risk adjustment. For example, obtaining mammograms is a process measure. Breast cancer related morbidity and mortality is the outcome of concern. The rate of obtaining mammograms in the appropriate population in a given practice is dependent on many factors including providers ordering the test, providers explaining the value of the test, the patient's pre-conceived beliefs of the value of the test, the ease of access to the test and the ability to pay for the test. Some of these factors seem almost entirely clinician controlled and others are almost entirely not clinician controlled, yet this is a very widely used process measure without adjustment.

Outcomes measures are likely to be the most meaningful metric. However, they are most likely to require some form of adjustment. A simple example is cancer treatment efficacy being adjusted for stage at presentation. Unfortunately, most adjustment is not so straightforward. Meaningful outcomes may also take years to show separation based upon the quality of care. A wrong site surgery has a fairly instantaneous outcome. The functional, behavioral, vocational and social outcomes related to pediatricians and family physicians screening for developmental disorders has a relatively long time horizon.

There are other ways to categorize quality measures. A very logical method to clinicians is division defined by *prevention, acute care or chronic disease management*. One would anticipate that a national evaluation would include all these types, but measurement of an individual provider may not include all three depending on the practice type. The Institute of Medicine defined six attribute domains of health care quality: *safe, timely, effective, efficient, equitable and patient-centered*. This creates an intellectual framework in measure development and selection. It also effectively addresses the need to consider attributes such as efficiency and equity that have not always been considered relevant by professionals focused on the single patient. The National Quality Strategy has translated this into six measurement domains listed as: *patient and family engagement, patient safety, care coordination, population/public health, efficient use of healthcare resources and clinical process/effectiveness*.

Quality measures may also be defined by the unit of measurement. There are obvious differences in numbers of members, patients or clinical events between a health plan, a hospital and an individual provider. But there is a more fundamental issue regarding *population* as compared to *patient*. Traditionally, clinicians have accepted responsibility for the care the clinician provided to the patient who came to the clinician for that care. As individual clinicians accept greater responsibility for populations, they are more and more measured on performance at the population level. It is not adequate to just do the right thing for the person in front of the clinician. Rather, the clinician or the team the clinician leads must make sure the patient receives the right care, even if that requires outreach and support provided outside of the context of a face to face encounter. The population of concern may vary greatly. It may be all the patients for a single clinician, or all the patients of an integrated healthcare system or even all the persons in a community. But the conceptual difference from a single patient focus is consistent. The transition from single patient focus to population management has many reasons. In some cases it is because clinicians have aggregated into healthcare delivery systems and seek to be evaluated or rewarded based upon efficacy of population management. The transition to value based payment has caused many to recognize that aggregation creates a larger patient population size being measured and thus spreads risk and reduces the potential for adverse effects based upon the randomness of results inherent in small population size. In other cases, it is because clinicians recognize their role in improving access, chronic condition management and other factors that justify population as a unit of measurement. While, population measures may be relatively irrelevant for those who provide time limited specialty acute care, such as an orthopedist who repairs a fractured hip, if that same orthopedist is part of a multi-specialty group that manages a population of persons with osteoarthritis, population based metrics may be valid. Consideration of population metrics also requires consideration of special populations or a range of populations. Measurement of our national healthcare requires a scope sufficient to measure care of different age segments, genders, races and ethnicities, socio-economic status and a host of other population subsets.

Measure Selection

There are several decision points that are undertaken in deciding what to measure. Some are alluded to above with respect to creating an appropriately broad scope of measures that relate to the key attributes of quality. Basics include the following:

1. The condition is meaningful to the population of concern.
2. There is a clearly defined measurable structure, process or outcome.
3. If not an outcome measure, there is an acceptable evidence base for the structure or process of care being related to an outcome.
4. There are existing opportunities for improvement based upon preliminary measurements. This may be due to regional or institutional variation or may be overall suboptimal performance across the population. These are often called gaps in care.
5. Measurement is feasible.
6. The cost and effort devoted to measurement is justified when balanced against the attention and resources that might otherwise be used in improving health.

Each one of these points raises issues. For example, an advocacy group may be justified in believing there should be national quality measures related to the disease that is their reason for existence, but others with a broader perspective may disagree. Those same parties with a broader perspective may conclude that not all measures must be for the most prevalent conditions and that especially vulnerable populations need a measurement focus. There may be controversy regarding the evidence. Should mammography start at 40 or 50? Should it be every year or every other year? What is "feasible" and "efficient" may vary depending upon the level of infrastructure or choices made in measure definitions. A claims based/administrative data based measure of quality may be useful and feasible, whereas chart audit may be superior, but wholly impractical, even if technically feasible. A measure that drives systems of care to change in a way that improves overall care for multiple conditions, not just the target condition, is ideal, whereas a measure that merely results in clinicians playing to the test is less desirable.

Denominators, Population Size and Attribution

Part of relevancy or being meaningful is frequency of the event or prevalence of the illness. But, prevalence also has a direct bearing on whether meaningful measurement can be accomplished. Having a large denominator in a measure has several advantages. The first is that the measure is now a "study" effectively powered to demonstrate real rather than random effects with some high degree of probability. The other advantage is that the probability of skew created by a subpopulation is less. This reduces the need to risk adjust or reduces the error inherent in the imperfections associated with risk adjustment. For example, it is possibly the case that two health plans of 100,000 members each in the same region can be so significantly different in member characteristics that this difference in characteristics would affect the probability of attaining certain results, but a significant difference in characteristics is substantially more likely when the comparison is between two single clinicians. This phenomenon has relevancy in determining the unit of measurement. It may seem desirable to compare two physicians for their ability to get a Hemoglobin A1c to goal. But that may well not be possible with any validity based upon the denominator of the measure. It is somewhat surprising how few patients with a specific condition many single clinicians have. This small number phenomenon is made worse when the measurement is by payer rather than aggregating the clinician's entire patient panel. An all payer measurement of a practice site may be more valid. Measurement of a collection of practice sites within an integrated healthcare delivery system may be even more legitimate.

Value based payment language requires measurement of an entity. How a patient is assigned to that entity varies. For a Medicare Advantage (Part C) plan, Medicare beneficiaries must enroll in a plan. Some the care they received or did not receive may not have been while a member of that plan, but the measurement year membership is clear. For example, a health plan will get credit for a screening colonoscopy paid for by another prior plan if done within the required look back time period. However, the measured plan must be able to demonstrate with records that it was performed. Likewise, if another plan failed to get the member to such screening for many years past the recommended performance date, the new plan is still responsible to fix the gap in care within the single measurement year.

In many cases attribution is not so simple. Patients often see many doctors, for example. Assume a patient has COPD and hypertension. Annually the patient sees a pulmonologist, who also seems to do a significant amount of primary care for other patients based simply upon billing/procedure codes submitted by the pulmonologist to a payer. Twice a year the patient sees a doctor, who is mutually acknowledged by the patient and that doctor to be the primary care physician, and receives a general assessment and blood pressure measurement. The patient experiences a burn on his arm one holiday weekend and has three visits to an urgent care facility for assessment and dressing changes. The doctor there is a family physician, but does not provide chronic care management or preventive services other than immunizations. The patient then manages the burn on his own. Attribution may assign this patient to the urgent care doctor as this doctor had the plurality of office visits performed on the member during the year. Of course, attribution could be different if the database and logic used was set up so that the urgent care physician could not have a patient attributed to him, except for assessment of the care she or he provided (e.g. a measure of the quality of minor burn care). Diagnoses could theoretically be used to define primary care, but this would be an extraordinary challenge given the breadth and overlap of conditions managed by different clinicians. However, diagnosis may be valid for assignment in the case of the clinician who reported the diagnosis of hypertension for the visit being assigned the responsibility of getting the blood pressure to the goal. The performance of a Medicare Annual Wellness Visit might be used to define the Medicare beneficiary's primary care clinician, but the Annual Wellness Visit may be performed by anyone, not just the primary care staff by current rules. Where this becomes especially relevant is when a population is to be managed and payment is based upon this. The managing clinicians may effectively manage someone who ultimately is not even attributed to them and potentially fail to manage someone who is ultimately attributed to them, but whom they thought was the responsibility of another entity.

As a general rule, assignment of responsibility for a quality metric should consider the locus of control of the party being measured. Control may not be complete. There may be patient factors. There may be system factors. These alone do not make measurement pointless. But performance is unlikely to improve and behavior unlikely to change if the result measured is entirely outside of the control of the provider of care being measured. A good example of this limitation is a measure of the national cost of care trends called the Sustainable Growth Rate (SGR). From a national economic perspective it is logical to assert that the segment of the economy devoted to healthcare expenditures cannot consistently grow faster than the overall economy. However, the SGR is enforced at the individual clinician level and is based upon cost trends at a national level of a subset of Medicare expenditures – those paid on the physician fee schedule. No amount of dedication to stewardship of resources by a single individual will have an impact on the SGR. But payment reductions when the SGR is exceeded fall upon every individual.

Adjustments

The perfectly fair adjustor that makes all comparisons valid is the Holy Grail. This is the domain of the statistical experts. Adjustment can create more valid comparisons. It also introduces an element that clinicians can perceive as invalid or obtuse. The greater the level of sophistication of the adjustment, the more complex it typically becomes and the more likely it will appear to be a "black box" to the party being measured. For most measures there is no accepted adjustor. Some bear mentioning, however. The most significant risk adjustment relates to payments to plans for populations. Medicare Advantage plans have been paid this way for quite some time and new exchange products will use a closely related adjustor to redistribute revenue between plans. The adjustment is the Centers for Medicare and Medicaid Services (CMS) Hierarchical Condition Category (HCC) system. This system is diagnosis based and does require that the diagnosis be managed, evaluated, assessed or treated, if it is to be included in the payment adjustment algorithm. Nonetheless, the huge financial impact of this adjustor and the response/need of plans to maximize revenue using it, has raised concerns that it is not just adjusting for risk related *expenditures*, but has become a major *revenue* center. This is an example of how risk adjustment may generate as much controversy as it resolves. There are methods to estimate probability of all cause readmission that are tested and being used (e.g., by the National Committee on Quality Assurance). The logic and specific mathematics of these models do not translate to other uses, such as adjusting for expected emergency department visit rates or expected rate of blood pressure being at goal.

Another commonly used adjustment is some form of outlier methodology. Outlier patients could be eliminated altogether. For example, one patient uses the emergency department 20 times a year and that one patient drives the emergency visit rate per patient for a practice. Another practice with the same number of patients has 20 patients who visit the emergency room once each. They have the same rate. However, it may be that the first practice has expanded hours, always immediately responds to pages and manages a wide range of conditions in the office, while the other practice has done little to reduce use of the emergency room as a site of the type of care that could be provided in the office. The outlier patient results in incorrect conclusions about the first office. A more typical method involves truncating outlier costs. A large group involved in a risk sharing arrangement will have costs of up to $100,000 per year for a given patient attributed to the group. Costs over this amount are not attributed. This reduces the effect of a single patient on per capita or per member per month expenses, but does not eliminate any recognition of the costs. Therefore, under this methodology, there is no chance that a $99,000 patient would appear more expensive than a $200,000 patient.

Episode treatment groups may be used to compare total costs of care for a specific condition. This method defines a condition and has rules as to when the condition starts and ends, i.e. when it is an episode. It also includes rules as to which expenses are condition related and which expenses are not condition related. Some models also divide related expenses into those that are expected and those that are complication related. An example of an episode treatment group would be the cost of care over a year for a patient with heart failure. It would start at the beginning of the year, even if the heart failure was not diagnosed until mid-year. All office visits to certain specialties would be included, even if the diagnosis on the claim was not heart failure. This would account for other potentially related conditions being included. Certain procedures such as echocardiograms, electrolyte and renal chemistries, cardiac catheterizations and cardiac rehabilitation would be included whereas care for a fracture of the radius would not be included. Certain inpatient diagnosis related groups would be included, whereas others would not. While this is simply intended as an example, it becomes obvious that a host of decisions must be made about what is or is not part of the episode. The radius fracture could be due to a fall caused by debility related to heart failure. The visit to the cardiologist may have been for dyspnea that was actually caused by anemia from a gastrointestinal blood loss and not remotely heart failure related. If costs are used for comparison purposes, there needs to be a decision as to how to handle price variation. This is especially important outside of Medicare where allowed payment amounts may vary considerably. If one seeks to measure real costs, then price variation may be relevant. For example, a group that accepts risk for the cost of care may save money without adversely affecting quality by simply using a lower cost provider such as a free standing radiology facility rather than a hospital based facility. On the other hand, if the goal is to look at efficiency related to utilization patterns, price may not be relevant and could actually obfuscate the analysis.

Propensity matching is used at times. This methodology looks at matching two populations through weighting methods. Then comparison is made. Again decisions need to be made about how weighting is made and what models are used for weighting. Would a historical average over the last 3 years be used to create prospective weights or would the activity of the measurement year be used to retroactively create weights?

Adjusting for socio-economic status (SES) is controversial. Few would dispute the social determinants of health such as wealth and education. However, adjusting for these might mean that it is acceptable to have lower quality of care for those in a lower SES. The debate about test performance in schools and the quality of the school is just this type of debate. It is not just a healthcare quality issue, but a broader social issue. What may determine the need to adjust or not is how the measurement is used. If safety net facilities are generally acknowledged as doing incredible work with challenging populations, yet a pay for performance system drives them into the red financially, there is a problem. The solutions to that problem may be less obvious, but may include a factor related to SES or comparison to peer entities at least. If the use is simply to create information for facilities to use over time, SES adjustment may be irrelevant.

Setting Goals and Thresholds

Various terms are used for a result that is desired. It could be a goal, i.e., something that is sought to be achieved. It could be a benchmark, which usually means a result that is excellent, possible and has been attained by some entity. It could be a threshold, meaning that attainment triggers something, such as additional payment. Each measure may have all of these and there may be multiple tiers or thresholds. The distinctions may be irrelevant if the goal of an organization is to hit the threshold.

A measure usually must be tested to determine if there are variations or gaps and if it can be reliably collected/performed. This testing process also allows an historically-based definition of a goal, median, threshold or top benchmark performance. It may be that the ideal is 100 % of the time XX will occur. But, as clinicians know, there are usually valid reasons for performance at a level of less than 100 %. This is why practice guidelines are called guidelines. There are reasons such as patient rights or other conditions that are too rare or diverse to list as exclusions that affect results. Therefore, historical norms and relative rates are typically used. The goal of measurement is first and foremost to drive *improvement*. So a practice or a hospital may focus on pushing the numbers in the desired direction. The public or a value conscious payer may be equally or more interested in identifying and/or rewarding higher *performance*. This potential dichotomy is characterized as pay for performance contrasted with pay for improvement, when payment is involved. The arguments for both methods are strong. Failing to recognize improvement can create hopelessness and disadvantage those who care for the most challenging populations. Rewarding improvement alone fails to recognize those who may have heavily invested in improvement long ago and now are sustaining those results. They may be improving, but in areas for which there are not yet measures used by the performance program. If improvement alone is recognized, they would be deemed failures because of their very success, whereas a perennial poor performer without legitimate explanation for past results finally improves a little and is now deemed the successful party. A hybrid method recognizing performance, but also recognizing improvement may be used to address both positions.

An example of the real world challenges of setting thresholds is seen in the Medicare Pioneer ACO program. The program uses a comparison of the specific ACO cost trend to trends in a national reference population of beneficiaries who are not in the ACO. Accordingly, a high performing ACO in a cost efficient region can fail as there are no savings, because they are efficient historically, even when their absolute costs (not cost trends) are well below national medians of other ACOs or non ACO aligned beneficiaries. This is true, even if the ACO performs better than its regional non ACO providers. Presumably, such better performance is ACO related and not related to regional variation. On the other hand, an ACO that has historically high costs in an historically high cost region shows some improvement, and while still relatively costly, is rewarded. This would be true even if the ACO did no better than the regional providers. Another analysis that relies upon comparison to the local community or a nearby community may show different results. The Pioneer ACO method compares trends. Therefore, if the two populations being compared do not dramatically change over the time periods from baseline to measurement, risk adjustment is less of an issue. So this method has some appeal. However, this method may cause one organization that is doing good work, to move away from an alternative payment method that is in theory designed to pay for value, because the organization is not being paid for the value it brings and is not recovering the investment costs necessary to obtain those results.

The intended use of the measure also defines how the thresholds should be set. The goal could be to reward only the top performers. In this case, the threshold is either purely performance relative to a pre-defined percentile (e.g. the top quartile) or attaining a result that based on history represents top performance. The latter may be selected so that a specific target can be announced in advance. However, the threshold would be different if all but low performers were to be recognized for investing in improvement. The threshold could also be a gate. For example, it may be that the structure of the program is to allow shared savings in cost of care for a population. However, the payer wants to be certain that quality did not deteriorate while savings were achieved. In this case, a floor quality performance rate might be the ticket to sharing savings. It could be that quality metrics must be maintained, but need not improve or be higher than the norm to pass through the gate for sharing in savings.

Where and how the dial is set also relates to other objectives. If the goal is to get providers to seriously think about measuring quality, one might just pay for reporting as was done in the CMS Physician Quality Reporting System (PQRS). If the goal is to drive lower performing providers out of the market and to force them to merge their entity with or lose their patients to an organization that has a formula for success, then targets may be rather aggressive. They may also need to be adjusted in a way that is local market dependent if high targets based on national norms would mean there were no providers left standing. The amount of money (if any) at stake may also determine the threshold of success. High performance reward thresholds may be set at a level of very high performance if the reward is unequivocally a bonus payment.

The same might be true if the target result was highly aspirational and what was at stake was a trophy. However, if the payment is essential for operations, it is unlikely a target that fatally wounds all but a few high performers could be chosen.

A by-product of setting performance goals based upon historical results is that measures should not be perpetually modified. Some stability and consistency is needed. There are other reasons for this such as the added costs of measurement if abstraction software must be constantly modified for ever changing measures.

Finally, thresholds may be selected based upon confidence intervals around a measure. In other words, the threshold is selected because it represents performance that is statistically highly likely not to be a random effect. Assume that the score 0.75 is the threshold result for the top quartile among a group of entities being measured. Assume 0.75 means 75 % of the time the desired process was performed and 1.0 means it occurred 100 % of the time. However, the individual entities being measured really have a result within the band of X plus or minus 0.25 with a 95 % probability based upon their population sizes. Assume the entities are similar in population and this confidence interval is constant. It would probably not be reasonable to conclude that threshold must be 1.0, even though only if the threshold is set at 1.0 can it be certain that the actual result is 0.75 or greater. It might be more reasonable to set the threshold at 0.5 knowing that all actual 0.75 performers and above will be recognized. This decision also means that entities that are actually only at 0.25 may also get recognized. If these alternatives are not acceptable, a minimum denominator that reduces the size of the confidence interval may be selected. However, this may exclude too may entities for the goal of the program. Ultimately, such a calculus and logic could result in abandonment of the measure as being useful or feasible.

Other Challenges

There are a host of other challenges in measurement and evaluation. Most healthcare expenses in Medicare are for beneficiaries with multiple chronic conditions. Most quality measures are single condition oriented. Those with expertise in caring for the multi-morbid recognize the weakness of such measurement. Recognition of weakness rises to serious concern when performance measures affect payment as is the case in the Value Based Purchasing provisions of the ACA. Care for those with multiple chronic illnesses requires clinician and patient to set priorities. The patient's values may direct that a goal that makes sense for other patients is not set as a goal for them. There are patient experience surveys that address whether the patient felt involved and respected in their care and such surveys may provide a mechanism to measure patient centeredness, which may be what matters most for this population. The Consumer Assessment of Healthcare Providers and Systems (CAHPS) program from the Agency for Healthcare Research and Quality (AHRQ) is designed to achieve measurement of patient-centeredness and is also expected to be part of Medicare evaluation programs.

There are not well defined measures for many provider types and population subsets that could be the dominant type of patient for a specific provider. Clinicians who care for a highly atypical patient population may not be appropriately measured by instruments that work well for those caring for the more typical population mix. At extremes, adjustment is likely to be ineffective in addressing this problem.

Performance measurement is intended to support quality care. It is important to acknowledge that while reducing variation in care using evidence based standards is generally desirable and likely to improve the health of a population, care must be applied at the individual patient level.

Developing Measures Through Consensus

Quality measures used within the ACA must meet certain standards. They are generally developed by using a process of consensus, endorsement and validation. The National Quality Forum (NQF) plays a major role in endorsing measures that have been developed and presently has a formal role in the PQRS process. It also may convene groups to develop measures and endorse measurement processes. Many organizations may develop measures, such as a medical specialty society, AHRQ or the National Committee on Quality Assurance (NCQA). Measures may be used in ways that are not exactly as intended in some programs (e.g. in a private payer program), but the use in ACA Value Based Payment programs is more tightly governed. These programs go through the rule making processes of the federal government with published proposed rules, comment and publication of final rules.

National Quality Strategy: Prioritization and Alignment

One serious concern is the proliferation of measures and measurement. In an ideal world, measurement would be organic in care, not just built into documentation systems. It would contribute to focusing on what really matters. Many clinicians using electronic records are all too familiar with the concern that record structure seems to support payment and reporting programs at the expense of supporting clinical care, patient interaction, clinician focus and critical thinking, even if the same clinician acknowledges the many merits of selected measurement and electronic records. There are legitimate concerns that the cost of measurement diverts resources that could be better used. The Institute of Medicine has labelled the need to combat measure proliferation as "Counting What Counts". The National Quality Strategy (NQS) is designed to address this as well. The measures and measurement of the ACA will reflect the NQS as amended periodically.

The National Quality Strategy was first published in 2011. It is led by the Agency for Healthcare Research and Quality (AHRQ) on behalf of the U.S. Department of Health and Human Services (HHS). It was established as part of the Affordable Care Act in order to facilitate a consistent focus on quality improvement efforts and a nationwide approach to measuring quality. The ACA requires HHS agencies to develop Agency-Specific Plans to achieve the NQS priorities; establish annual benchmarks for success; and regularly report on progress against these benchmarks.

The ACA also established the Interagency Working Group on Health Care Quality. This group includes 24 Federal agencies and has a mission to foster collaboration, cooperation, and consultation on quality-related efforts between Federal departments and agencies, and with the private sector. The NQS is not a federal program despite the essential facilitation role federal agencies play and the requirements of the ACA to have a national strategy. The NQS achieves its goal by working with the NQF. It has two formal partnerships: the National Priorities Partnership and the Measures Application Partnership. The National Priorities Partnership is made up of over 50 national organizations with a shared vision to achieve better health, and a safe, equitable, and value-driven healthcare system. The Measures Application Partnership is a public-private partnership that reviews performance measures for potential use in Federal public reporting and performance-based payment programs. It also seeks to align measures used in public and private payer programs.

Project evaluations, such as those of new activities of the Center for Medicare and Medicaid Innovation (CMMI) will have evaluation metrics relevant to the specific project. However, major programs such as Medicare 5 Star, PQRS and other Value Based Purchasing programs will reflect these activities. Programs such as PQRS, Meaningful Use and others will align as the NQS achieves its goals. The NQS 2013 Progress Report to Congress outlines measures related to the six priorities (Table 9.1).

Table 9.1 NQS - Improving Quality Across Six Priority Areas (2013 Report to Congress)

Measure focus	Measure name/description
Priority 1. Making care safer by reducing harm caused in the delivery of care	
Hospital-acquired conditions	Incidence of measurable hospital-acquired conditions
Hospital readmissions	All-payer 30-day readmission rate
Priority 2. Ensuring that each person and family is engaged as partners in their care	
Timely care	Adults who needed care right away for an illness, injury, or condition in the last 12 months who sometimes or never got care as soon as wanted
Decision making	People with a usual source of care whose health care providers sometimes or never discuss decisions with them
Priority 3. Promoting effective communication and coordination of care	
Patient-centered medical home	Percentage of children needing care coordination who receive effective care coordination
3-Item care transition measure ®	During this hospital stay, staff took my preferences and those of my family or caregiver into account in deciding what my health care needs would be when I left
	When I left the hospital, I had a good understanding of the things I was responsible for in managing my health
	When I left the hospital, I clearly understood the purpose for taking each of my medications

(continued)

Table 9.1 (continued)

Measure focus	Measure name/description
Priority 4. Promoting the most effective prevention and treatment practices for the leading causes of mortality, starting with cardiovascular disease	
Aspirin use	Outpatient visits at which adults with cardiovascular disease are prescribed/maintained on aspirin
Blood pressure control	Adults with hypertension who have adequately controlled blood pressure
Cholesterol management	Adults with high cholesterol who have adequate control
Smoking cessation	Outpatient visits at which current tobacco users received tobacco cessation counseling or cessation medications
Priority 5. Working with communities to promote wide use of best practices to enable healthy living	
Depression	Percentage of adults who reported symptoms of a major depressive episode in the last 12 months who received treatment for depression in the last 12 months
Obesity	Proportion of adults who are obese
Priority 6. Making quality care more affordable for individuals, families, employers, and governments by developing and spreading new health care delivery models	
Out-of-pocket expenses	Percentage of people under 65 with out-of-pocket medical and premium expenses greater than 10 % of income
Health spending per capita	Annual all-payer health care spending per person

Specific measures within specific federal programs are too numerous to list. For example, the 2014 Medicare Part C 5 Star program has 36 measures and the Part D 5 Star program has 15 measures. PQRS has hundreds because it is for use by many different professional disciplines. ACOs must report 33 quality measures in the Medicare Shared Savings Program.

Summary

Society, government and professionals have devoted considerable time and effort to devising methods to improve care and achieve the goals of the Triple Aim. It is a work in progress. There is a mandate in the ACA to measure, improve measurement and use measurement of value in payment. The efficacy of these efforts will be a measure of the success of the ACA itself.

Chapter 10
Targeting Interventions and Populations

Adam G. Golden, Michael A. Silverman, and Thomas T.H. Wan

The Need for Geriatric-Focused Models of Care

Medically complex older adults are at high risk for receiving costly and fragmented care from health care professionals who are often unfamiliar with the prior evaluation of their medical and psychosocial issues [1]. Failure to provide effective care coordination may result in exposure to potentially dangerous procedures, excessive use of medications, and unnecessary transitions in care between inpatient, outpatient and long-term care facilities. Unnecessary transitions in care may expose patients to serious nosocomial infections and increase the risk of iatrogenic events, geriatric syndromes (i.e. falls, delirium, pressure ulcers, urinary incontinence), and functional dependency [2, 3].

In other cases, the lack of care coordination may prevent patients from receiving services that they need. For example, many seniors may not have the appropriate

---

Disclosure Drs. Golden and Wan received support from the National Institute on Minority Health and Health Disparities of the National Institutes of Health under Award Number U24MD006954. The content is solely the responsibility of the authors and does not necessarily represent the official views of the National Institutes of Health.

A.G. Golden, M.D., M.B.A. (✉)
Department of Internal Medicine, University of Central Florida College of Medicine, Orlando Veterans Affairs Medical Center, 5201 Raymond Street, Orlando, FL 32803, USA
e-mail: adam.golden@ucf.edu

M.A. Silverman, M.D., M.P.H.
Geriatrics & Extended Care, West Palm Beach Veterans Affairs Medical Center,
7305 North Military Trail, Riviera Beach, FL 33410-7417, USA

T.T.H. Wan, Ph.D.
College of Health and Public Affairs, University of Central Florida,
4000 Central Florida Blvd, Orlando, FL 32816-3680, USA

services and equipment to live at home which puts them at-risk for issues such as self-neglect or preventable falls. The implementation of home-based support services may also prevent cases of nursing home institutionalization.

Complicating matters is the fact that Medicare does not provide many services that are vital to frail older adults (i.e. long-term care, home health aides). The services provided to Medicare Advantage beneficiaries may decrease as this entitlement faces increased austerity measures under the *ACA*.

The Target Population

The terms "vulnerable," "at-risk," "dependent," and "frail" are often used to describe the segment of older adults who are high utilizers of health care resources. Although all four terms have specific research definitions, the clinical picture involves people of with one or more of the following characteristics listed in Table 10.1.

These issues are often interrelated and increase in prevalence with advanced age [4]. Of great concern is the fact that persons 85 years of age and older continue to be the fastest growing segment of the population. Functional and cognitive impairments place this segment of the older adult population at a relatively higher risk for nursing home placement. Not surprisingly, the prevalence of nursing home placement increases from 2 % among older adults age 65–74 to 20 % among those 85 years of age and older [5].

While many older adults have no serious health issues, 24 % have four or more chronic medical conditions and half have one or more geriatric syndromes [6]. Among Medicare beneficiaries, the total costs of care increase proportionally with the number of chronic medical conditions [7]. These medically complex elderly patients are also at a higher risk for hospitalization and are more vulnerable to iatrogenic complications during an acute care episode [3, 8].

Psychosocial issues may also define those "at risk." The smaller size and fragmented nature of modern families means that many older adults will not have adequate caregiver support at home. The increasing need for women to seek gainful

Table 10.1 Characteristics of older adults who are high utilizers of health care resources

Advanced progressive illness(es)
Declining ability to perform activities of daily living (i.e. toileting, bathing, dressing, eating, transferring)
Declining ability to perform instrumental activities of daily living (i.e. using a telephone, cooking a meal, balancing a checkbook)
Cognitive impairment
Presence of one or more geriatric syndromes (i.e. falls, polypharmacy, unintentional weight loss, incontinence, falls, and pressure ulcers)
Hearing and vision impairment

employment has further complicated the efforts of many families to provide adequate home-based caregiver support.

Indigent older adults who qualify for both Medicare and Medicaid entitlements are estimated to number approximately nine million and cost federal and state governments $250 billion annually [9]. The per capita health care costs for these "dual eligible" beneficiaries is five times higher than age-sex matched Medicare enrollees [10]. Other older adults with limited financial resources do not meet the strict criteria to qualify for Medicaid. Many cannot afford community-based or long-term care services that are provided for free to Medicaid beneficiaries.

Identifying High Risk Populations

Geriatric health care programs often report anecdotal cases of older adults who dramatically improved as a result of a specific intervention. However, demonstrating the evidence-based benefit of geriatric interventions has often been difficult to accomplish. Given the limited resources of the modern health care system, the key objective for any geriatric-focused program is to develop specific interventions that target the appropriate patient population at the appropriate time. The "appropriate" population is one for whom an intervention would likely have a significant impact (Table 10.2). If the target population is too healthy, the patients will be at a lower risk for adverse events. As such, finite health care resources would be misdirected toward patients for whom the potential impact of a geriatric intervention would be very limited.

On the opposite end of the spectrum, there are patients who are not likely to benefit from interventions due to declining health or the presence of severe functional or cognitive impairments. In these cases, resources would be wasted providing geriatric interventions to patients with a limited chance for improvement. Identifying the appropriate target population will vary depending on the specific geriatric intervention.

Several screening tools have been developed to rapidly identify "at-risk" older adults. The Probability of Repeated Admission score (Pra) is a short self-administered screening tool that was developed to identify community-dwelling older adults at high risk for hospital admission. A recent review of the Pra score found that this

Table 10.2 Potential factors to measure in the assessment of geriatric-focused interventions	Quality of life
	Health care costs (Medicare, Medicaid)
	Hospital admission and readmission
	Nursing home placement
	Functional impairment
	Presence of geriatric syndromes
	Caregiver burden

screening tool identifies patients at high risk for hospitalization [11]. However it is not reliable at identifying low risk patients. Screening tools that have been validated for use in a telephone-based interview (i.e. Telephone Interview for Cognitive Status, AD8) may aid in the assessment of homebound and geographically isolated older adults [12].

Other assessment tools use computer software to analyze databased information to estimate risk among patients of a specific population. The Care Assessment Need (CAN) score is used by the Veterans Health Administration to estimate the probability of hospital admission and/or death within a 90-day and 1-year period [13]. Patients with the highest score have a 72 % probability of either hospital admission or death within 1 year. The Elder Risk Assessment was developed at the Mayo Clinic to estimate risk of hospitalization, hip fracture, and emergency department use among older adult outpatients [14]. The DxCG risk score uses age, gender, and medical claims information to predict resource utilization [15].

A review of nine screening tools used to assess the risk of poor outcomes in older inpatients found that only the Identification of Seniors at Risk (ISAR) score predicted mortality, institutionalization, readmission, and health care resource use [16]. Not included in the review was the Transitional Care Model Screening Criteria. This ten-item tool for hospitalized older adults has been shown to identify those patients who will have a poor outcome during the post-discharge period [17].

In addition, many states have developed tools to identify older adults who meet the financial and medical criteria to qualify for Medicaid long-term care services. These tools may identify patients with functional impairments, chronic illnesses, cognitive impairments, and geriatric syndromes. These tools are also used to determine care management reimbursements for home- and community-based care. Even with such tools, the determination as to whether these patients need nursing home care or could remain at home with home- and community-based services often remains unclear due to the complex interactions among patients' nursing needs and psychosocial issues.

With limitations in resources it is also essential that geriatric-focused interventions demonstrate their ability to decrease health care costs and improve quality. Table 10.2 lists the general categories of factors that can be measured in the assessment of geriatric interventions. Over the course of a decade, Rand Health developed the Assessing Care for Vulnerable Elders (ACOVE) Project which identified specific quality indicators for 26 conditions that are prevalent in the older adult population [18].

Geriatric Care Models: Opportunities and Limitations

Unfortunately, there is currently no evidence-based consensus as to the proper models that will provide the most cost effective health care for the heterogeneous "at-risk" older adult population. As opposed to health care efforts involving children or young adults, this segment of the older adult population is extremely heterogeneous with regards to medical illnesses, functional impairment, physiological reserve, and psychosocial issues. Research studies of geriatric-focused intervention models reveal decreased hospitalization rates, quality of care, and health-care expenditures in some, but not all studies [8, 19–22].

Identifying the key features from these studies that might improve quality or lower costs is difficult because geriatric care models are highly heterogeneous with regard to reimbursement, patient selection, staff training, local health care practices, and care processes [23]. Furthermore, specific components of these details are often not provided in a research article. Improved outcomes in a research study may not be generalizable to patients receiving care through community-based medical systems. In fact, research studies of community-based geriatric interventions often exclude patients that may be at high risk for adverse outcomes. Patients who are non-English speakers, lack decision-making capacity, lack a caregiver, lack a telephone, or refuse to sign an informed consent are often excluded from research protocols [24].

Disease management programs have been shown to improve compliance with evidence-based guidelines and health care outcomes in adults with diabetes mellitus, congestive heart failure, and chronic obstructive pulmonary disease. The potential evidence-based benefits of such programs often do not apply to those older adults with significant comorbidities and limited life expectancy [24].

Disease Management models also place great emphasis on patient accountability to "take responsibility for their own health care." Such an emphasis may be reasonable for the general population, but is not a realistic option for many older adults. Dementia and cognitive impairments may make it difficult to remember recent and remote medical history. This same age group also has a high prevalence of hearing and vision impairment which makes communication with health care providers difficult. Language barriers and low health literacy may prevent patients from fully comprehending the details of the complex care that they are receiving. Still others may not able to provide health information to health care professionals due to an acute illness that affects the level of alertness.

Health Information Technology-Based Interventions

Electronic Health Record (EHR)

The EHR has emerged as a means for health care professionals to document and retrieve patient health care information at any time. EHR mitigates the problems due to lost or illegible paper charts. Most EHR systems have automated features that allow the provider to manage individual patients as well as panels of patients (i.e. health maintenance reminders, notification of abnormal laboratory values, and alerts for potential drug-drug interactions).

The potential opportunities and challenges associated with EHR are listed in Table 10.3. Initial studies have demonstrated improved guideline compliance and a

Table 10.3 Opportunities and challenges of the electronic medical record

Opportunities
Availability of patient health information at any time and location
Improved legibility
Decreased risk for lost or misplaced charting
Potential to decrease inappropriate testing, procedures, and hospitalizations
Integration of clinical decision support software
Improved ability to monitor quality
Ease of large scale outcomes studies
Challenges
Cost savings not proven
Poor interface among different health care systems/practices
Decreased physician efficiency
Interference with the doctor-patient relationship
Patient privacy concerns
"Note bloat"

lower risk of medication errors. These benefits are largely attributed to the use of clinical decision support and electronic provider order entry features [25].

Despite the theoretical and anecdotal benefits of decreasing the inappropriate duplication of health care resources, definitive outcomes studies have been inconclusive [26, 27]. The costs to install an EHR, train staff, and maintain the system is expensive and may outweigh any cost savings [27]. Studies that look at the pre- and post-implementation of EHRs on costs and quality of care may be limited by confounding factors due to concurrent care management and other system transitional care system changes [28].

In many cases, the EHR between different medical systems are not integrated. For community-based care managers, access to the medical records may be more difficult with each medical center and post-acute facility having a different password protected EHR [23]. Difficulty accessing and navigating EHR will also hamper health professional education, where clinical rotations may span only several weeks in duration.

Primary care physicians evaluating the diverse problems of medically complex elderly patients are especially vulnerable to the inefficiencies of EHR utilization. Much of the information in the electronic notes are there to satisfy quality improvement and billing documentation rather than the patients-specific clinical issues. As a result, it is more difficult for treating physicians to fill out these EHR templates that contain large amounts of unnecessary verbiage ("note bloat") [29] and to find significant clinical information. Time is also lost waiting to log into the EHR and to navigate through the system.

Slowing the physician's productivity could have a negative impact on income and physician job satisfaction. Since the physician's time with patients is fixed, the extra time typing and navigating the EHR takes away from direct patient care. The physician's eye-contact toward the computer, rather than the patient, damages the physician-patient relationship [30].

Telehealth (E-Health)

In theory, home telehealth (E-health) allows care managers to use evidence-based disease management strategies for patients with advanced chronic illnesses, such as diabetes, chronic obstructive pulmonary disease, and congestive heart failure. Home monitoring, including direct uploading of patient-specific physiologic and home data to the EHR, can allow for a potential early intervention before the patient's clinical deterioration requires emergent care. Telehealth is an appealing intervention for homebound and rural older adults. Interest in developing telehealth programs has been historically limited by the lack of reimbursement for non-face-to-face encounters. With implementation of the ACA, capitated payment models will provide new incentives to explore telehealth interventions.

Efforts to study the impact of telehealth on mortality, hospitalization and emergency department use have often yielded negative or inconclusive results [31]. The results of home telehealth studies are difficult to generalize due to the heterogeneity of technology modalities and devices as well as variation in patient characteristics [32]. Many lack a rigorous assessment of quality, accessibility, and cost. Without control groups, it remains unclear how much of an effect was due to the care coordination component of the disease management program rather than the home telehealth monitoring. More recently, the use of home telemonitoring for older patients with multiple health issues did not lower the rate of hospital admissions or emergency department visits [33].

Geriatric Evaluation and Management

The ability to improve outcomes of "at-risk" older adults through a "interdisciplinary" comprehensive geriatric assessment has become the cornerstone of geriatric health professional training. The ability of geriatricians acting alone to provide care that is of higher quality and more cost effective than primary care physicians has not been demonstrated [34]. The interdisciplinary comprehensive geriatric assessment involves an evaluation to identify and manage all significant medical illnesses, psychosocial issues, functional disabilities, and geriatric syndromes. Platforms for performing such evaluations include both inpatient and outpatient settings. Despite much heterogeneity in design, these models involve a direct clinical assessment by a nurse, physician, social worker, pharmacist, and rehabilitation therapist (physical, occupational, and/or speech). The evaluation involves the use of standardized assessment tools. The management component involves the implementation of a care plan that incorporates best practice strategies.

An analysis of both inpatient and outpatient VA Geriatric Evaluation and Management (GEM) programs by Cohen et al. showed no significant effects on survival [35]. The outpatient evaluation was able to demonstrate improvements in mental health and the inpatient evaluation was associated with reductions in functional decline.

A review of studies involving inpatient comprehensive geriatric assessments reveals that this intervention was associated with improved mortality, lower functional decline and a lower risk of nursing home placement compared to usual hospital care [36]. Many of these studies were conducted quite some time ago. In recent years, the implementation of quality measures and improvements in geriatric health profession education have increased the baseline standard hospital practice. Whether inpatient geriatric interventions can still provide significant benefits remains unclear as rates of delirium, falls, and functional decline remain high due to a high floor effect [37]. D'Souza and Gupta recently highlighted the fact that comprehensive geriatric assessments and geriatric-focused care management has not been shown to improve mortality or reduce hospital admissions [38].

Comprehensive Clinical Care Models

Accountable Care Organizations (ACOs)

Attempts to develop care coordination models that are cost-effective and provide high quality service have been plagued by the financial incentives of a fee-for-service system that rewards physician and medical center productivity. ACOs are provider network involving physicians, hospital, and/or health plans that are organized to deliver low cost, high quality care for panels of at least 5,000 Medicare patients. Participant networks have the opportunity to receive extra money if they can decrease Medicare costs below specific benchmarks and meet specific quality of care measures. The "shared savings" for the network provides a strong incentive to develop seamless communication among health care professionals across sites using an electronic health record. The program will also rely on care-coordination and disease management strategies to prevent unnecessary hospitalizations and emergency room visits. ACOs differ from an HMO as ACOs are not receiving capitated payments. Patients not required to stay in ACO network. As such, going "out-of-network" does not increase the patient's out-of-pocket costs.

After a tenfold increase in the number of ACOs between 2010 and 2013, the number of new ACO applications has slowed [39]. Further voluntary participation by new provider networks remains limited as the financial rewards remain uncertain compared to fee-for-service care.

There is currently much heterogeneity in the structure and processes of these organizations. More than half do not have a participating hospital [39]. Compared to non-ACO patients, those covered by an ACO were more likely to be at least 80 years of age and higher incomes [39]. They were also less likely to be covered by Medicaid or disabled.

Accountable Care Organizations (ACOs) have not consistently shown to save money or decrease the risk of rehospitalization in vulnerable older adults [40]. A major disincentive is that the initial costs (for integrated electronic medical records, staff retraining, etc.) may be significantly more than the potential savings [41, 42]. In addition, the potential loss of income to health care systems as a result of decreased hospital admissions may be a disincentive for hospital participation with ACOs. Establishing best practices for ACOs with regard to patient selection and care processes is needed to garner further support to develop new provider networks.

Patient-Centered Medical Home Model

In response to the current fragmented model of health care, the concept of the patient-centered medical home has arisen. This model is an approach to providing comprehensive primary care. The general principles of this model are listed in Table 10.4 [43]. These principles are quite familiar to geriatricians, but the medical home model has not consistently demonstrated a decrease in costs or in the utilization of hospital, emergency department, or ambulatory care services [44, 45]. Analyses of a statewide multipayer medical home model involving 32 primary care practices found that the medical home model was able to lower costs and hospitalizations only in patients with a high DxCG risk score [15, 45].

In a health care system where primary care physicians are relatively underpaid compared to their subspecialty colleagues, enthusiasm for physicians to participate in a medical home model may be limited unless they perceive clear financial advantages or improvements in their work environment. Similarly, many regions currently face shortages of primary care physicians which further inhibit the model's widespread implementation. For geriatricians caring for frail older adults, these principles make sense logically, but are often difficult to implement in the real world setting.

More recently, new legislation has been proposed to develop the *Better Care Program* [46]. This program would provide a flat fee to providers to coordinate care for older adults with multiple chronic conditions.

Table 10.4 Principles of a patient-centered medical home model	
	Personal physician
	Physician-directed interprofessional medical practice
	Whole person orientation (providing for all the patient's health care needs)
	Coordinated care across entire spectrum of care
	Emphasis on quality and patient safety
	Enhanced access

Concierge Medicine

Patient-centered, comprehensive, longitudinal care could also be provided through concierge medicine. The patient pays the physician directly for specified services and increased physician access. This model provides physicians with an economic incentive to deliver more personal care and expanded personal access to a smaller panel of patients. Patients who are "most vulnerable," those with limited financial resources and caregiver support, would be least likely to utilize this out-of-pocket model. In fact, any migration of primary care physicians toward more lucrative concierge practices could further lower the availability of primary care physicians for medically complex older adults.

PACE

The Program for All-Inclusive Care of the Elderly (PACE) was developed as a clinical model to provide community-based comprehensive and coordinated longitudinal care for dual-eligible older adults who meet the medical criteria for nursing home placement. PACE programs receive a capitated Medicare and Medicaid reimbursement and are responsible for all of the patient's medical and long-term care needs. The program provides transportation for patients to a centralized adult day care setting. At the day care, patients are evaluated and treated by an interdisciplinary team of health care professionals who are either employed or contracted to work with the PACE.

This model has been shown to decrease hospitalization rates and total Medicare costs [47, 48]. The interpretation of these results must be done with caution as there may be a selection bias among patients who elect to enroll in PACE versus those who receive services through other community-based Medicaid waiver programs [49]. The PACE physician is responsible for providing and coordinating all care for PACE enrollees. Thus, patients who require complex specialty care or have a positive long-term relationship with their specialist physicians may be less likely to enroll in this program [49].

At the state level, PACE programs provide care to only a very small number of homebound indigent older adults. In the state of Florida, for example, there were 725 patients enrolled in PACE compared with an expected enrollment of over 90,000 in the Statewide Medicaid Managed Care Long-term Care Program [50]. *Despite savings to Medicare, Medicaid reimbursements are 86 % higher than projected fee-for-service estimates* [47]. Similarly, the state of Florida estimates higher costs to Medicaid for enrollees in PACE compared to its Managed Care Long-Term Care Program which cares for patients that are on average older and frailer [50].

PACE models require a large amount of start-up capital to assemble the required services, necessitating support from large healthcare systems, or states. The concept has been around for many decades, but adoption of new PACE programs has been relatively slow, suggesting a modest return on investment.

Geriatric Resource for Assessment and Care of Elders (GRACE)

The GRACE model involves the efforts of both an advanced registered nurse practitioner and a social worker [51] to provide geriatric home assessments and care management to indigent older adult patients. These two health professionals meet with the patient's primary care provider and consult with an interdisciplinary team to develop an outpatient care plan and coordinate transitions in care. *Hospital admission rates were lower in the group at the highest risk* (as measured by the Pra) [52].

Hospice and Palliative Care

The Medicare hospice benefit has been shown to increase quality of life for patients with terminal illnesses. However, the cost savings of hospice versus fee-for-service Medicare remains unclear. Although high cost procedures and hospitalizations are avoided in some cases, hospice agencies bill Medicare at a daily rate over the course of months for many patients with limited end-of-life care needs. There is a well-documented correlation between the proliferation of for-profit hospice agencies and the increase in the number of patients receiving extended care under Hospice [53–55]. Much of this perceived overuse was noted among nursing home residents with a diagnosis of advanced dementia and failure to thrive. In this setting, the facility provides for all of the patient's custodial care needs, but the hospice agency is still able to bill at the full daily rate.

To qualify for hospice, patients must have a prognosis of less than 6 months. With the exception of end-stage cancers, it is difficult to predict 6 month life-expectancy in patients with an advanced illness [56]. Survival statistics for large group of patients may exist, but a reliable prediction for individuals, especially for those with end-stage dementia, is often not possible. In almost two-thirds of cases, physicians are overly optimistic in their prognosis of patients with advanced illness [57, 58]. In fact, Christakis et al. noted that the longer the relationship between the physician and the patient, the worse the accuracy of prognosis [57].

In contrast to the Medicare benefit of hospice, palliative care is an "approach" that is not dependent on life-expectancy of less than 6 months. Palliative care places greater emphasis on communication more than testing and procedures. There is a strong focus on clarifying patient-centered goals of treatment and addressing patient "suffering" (physical symptoms, mood disorders, spiritual and psychosocial concerns). Patients who receive a palliative care consult are more likely to set goals of care with staff, have improved family satisfaction, are less likely to go to ICU, and undergo less diagnostic and laboratory testing [59].

Defining patients that would most benefit from outpatient palliative care services might involve focusing on those with an end-stage illness or a very high score on a screening tool such as the CAN [13]. Such services should emphasize quality of life symptoms and define patient-centered goals of care. A major barrier to providing appropriate end-of-life care involve patient expectations. Many patients have difficulty accepting a poor prognosis and expect aggressive high-cost care. In a cohort of N = 10,000 patients with stage 4 lung cancer or colorectal cancer. Sixty-nine percent of lung and 81 % of CR cancer patients thought chemotherapy might be curative [60]. Capitated models need to be careful that their efforts to steer patients toward hospice and palliative care are not perceived as financially driven "death panels."

Home and Community-Based Medicaid Waivers

Most states have one or more Medicaid care coordination programs designed to identify and provide the services needed to delay or prevent institutionalization of dependent older adults. These programs are viewed by Medicaid as a cheaper alternative to the high cost of nursing home placement. Initial care coordination efforts focused on the ability of care managers to link dependent older adults with the fee-for-service resources needed to keep them at home. More recent care coordination programs place an increased emphasis on capitated payments to care management providers who would assume the risk of institutional nursing home care.

Data on cost savings is difficult to assess due to the large variability in program design, patient selection, and local availability of home-based health care resources [61]. Changing requirements, processes, and reimbursements adds further difficulty to measuring the longitudinal effectiveness of these programs.

Rather than preventing high cost nursing home care, some health policy experts raise an alarm that efforts to further expand home- and community-based programs will increase total Medicaid long-term care liabilities. The term "woodwork effect" describes the concern that much of the spending for community-based services will go toward the care of older adults who are at low risk for nursing home placement [62]. Medicaid would in effect pay for services that are already provided by the beneficiary's caregiver(s).

The woodwork effect would assume that the care needs of the Medicaid beneficiaries receiving home- and community-based services are substantially lower than among those who require institutional care [63]. However, screening criteria that can differentiate which frail older adults would be better served through home- and community-based services does not exist. In many cases, the decision regarding institutional versus home-based long-term care is based on complex psychosocial issues and the local referral patterns of hospitals and skilled nursing facilities [64].

A similar concern is noted in the use of Medicare resources for post-acute care. The utilization of skilled home care services has been shown to be a major source of the geographic variation in Medicare spending (even after adjusting for patient demographics, health status, and regional cost of living) [65].

It remains difficult to measure the care needs of nursing home residents compared to those receiving home and community-based services. Nursing home assessments regarding issues such as dementia-related behaviors and incontinence are based on the multi-day observation of an interdisciplinary team of health care professionals. Standardized assessments are performed using the Minimum Data Set (MDS) 3.0. Home assessments are based on care management assessments that often involve a one-time visit and a discussion with the caregiver.

Transitional Care Interventions

Up to 20 % of all Medicare beneficiaries who are admitted to the hospital are readmitted within 30 days [66]. Ninety-eight percent involve beneficiaries with multiple chronic illnesses [67]. The majority of these readmissions are potentially preventable. As such, Medicare resources are being wasted and patients are being exposed to further iatrogenic risks.

In response, the ACA allocated $500 million for the Community-Based Care Transitions Program. This program will test models for improving care transitions from the hospital to other settings and reducing readmissions of high-risk Medicare beneficiaries [68]. Currently based at 102 sites around the country, the goal of this program is to establish best practices that can lower rehospitalizations rates by 20 %.

Transitional Care Model (TCM)

TCM is designed to provide for the coordination and delivery of care for hospitalized older adults who are at high risk for poor outcomes on discharge. The program utilizes an advance practice nurse who is involved in the discharge planning process and provides two months of post-discharge home visit and telephone follow-up. Multiple studies have shown a decrease in rehospitalizations and health care costs with this intervention [69].

Transitional Care for Nursing Home Residents

Implementing transitional care initiatives in the long-term care setting is an uphill battle as there are strong financial incentives for hospitals, physicians, and nursing homes to shuffle elderly patients back and forth between acute and long-term care facilities [64, 70]. Likewise, nursing homes are financially disincentivized to provide high cost medical care.

INTERACT is a recent quality improvement program designed to reduce potentially avoidable nursing home hospitalizations [71]. INTERACT involves strategies to assist nursing home staff in the early identification, assessment, communication, and documentation of changes in resident status. The program also involves strategies for improved care planning and use of hospice and palliative care. The INTERACT II study reported a 17 % decrease in hospital admissions with greater reductions among facilities with more active participation in the program [72]. A more recent study using INTERACT found a similar association between higher nursing home participation and lower rates of potentially avoidable hospitalizations [73]. The amount of reduction, however, was not statistically significant.

Transitioning from the Long-Term Care Facility to "Home"

Another focus of transitional care efforts is to provide the resources needed for long-term care residents to return to the community. Medically complex patients and those with inadequate caregiver support are more likely to need post-acute care [74]. Following the US Supreme Court's 1999 decision in Olmstead versus L.C. [75], most states have developed Medicaid programs to transition nursing home residents back into the community. Best practice models do not exist. The effectiveness of these programs is dependent on many variables including the local availability of resources, such as assisted living facilities, home care agencies, and Medicaid waiver slots.

The longer the person remains in the long-term care facility, the more difficult it will be to transition the older adult back into the community. By providing assistance with ADLs to residents, nursing homes can foster an environment of "learned dependency" [23]. In addition, many residents have had to sell their home and possessions which complicates nursing home discharge efforts.

Conclusion

In a fee-for-service system, strong financial incentives exist among physicians, hospitals, and long-term care facilities to provide a high volume of care [64, 76]. These incentives have limited the effectiveness of many geriatric-focused interventions. Often overlooked is the impact on physician efficiency and reimbursement. The true impact of geriatric-focused interventions to lower health care costs and improve quality will not likely occur unless the patient belongs to a capitated payment program or is in an integrated care delivery system that provides significant financial incentives to decrease health care costs.

The implementation of ACOs represents an important step in this direction. Of potentially greater impact is the Center for Medicare & Medicaid Innovation's (CMMI) funding of the Bundled Payment for Care Improvement (BPCI) Initiative. The purpose of this initiative is to measure the potential impact of a single ("bundled") for an entire episode of care. The bundle could include the hospital, physician fees, post-acute care, and 30 day rehospitalization costs.

Identifying the "best" geriatric interventional model is not the right question to ask. Because of the medical and psychosocial heterogeneity of the vulnerable older adult population, it is likely that health systems will need to develop an array of services that can most closely meet the needs of the individual patient [49]. The evaluation of these models will require a conceptually grounded approach with rigorous study design.

References

1. Golden AG, Mintzer MJ, Silverman MA. Uncovering a "new" clinical niche for the geriatrician. Ann Long-Term Care Clin Care Aging. 2013;21(6):21–2.
2. Creditor MC. Hazards of hospitalization of the elderly. Ann Intern Med. 1993;118(3):219–23.
3. Covinsky KE, Pierluissi E, Johnston CB. Hospitalization associated disability: "she was probably able to ambulate, but I'm not sure". JAMA. 2011;306(16):1782–93.
4. Wan TTH, Breen JM, Zhang NJ, Unruh L. Improving the quality of care in nursing homes. Baltimore: Johns Hopkins University Press; 2010.
5. Kane RL, Ouslander JG, Abrass IB, Resnick B. The geriatric patient: demography, epidemiology, and health services utilization. In: Essentials of clinical geriatrics. 7th ed. New York: McGraw Hill; 2013.
6. Cigolle CT, Langa KM, Kabeto MV, Tian Z, Blaum CS. Geriatric conditions and disability: the Health and Retirement Study. Ann Intern Med. 2007;147(3):156–64.
7. Dobson A, DaVanzo JE, Heath S, Shimer M, Berger G, Pick A, et al. Medicare payment bundling: insights from claims data and policy implications. American Hospital Association and Association of American Medical Colleges. 2012. http://www.aha.org/content/12/ahaaamcbundlingreport.pdf
8. Gillick MR. When frail elderly adults get sick: alternatives to hospitalization. Ann Intern Med. 2014;160(3):201–2.
9. Congressional Budget Office. Dual-eligible beneficiaries of Medicare and Medicaid: characteristics, health care spending and evolving policies [Internet]. 2013. http://www.cbo.gov/sites/default/files/cbofiles/attachments/44308_DualEligibles.pdf. [Cited January 18, 2014].
10. Lyons B, Watts MO. Health reform opportunities: improving policy for dual eligible [Internet]. Washington, DC: Kaiser Family Foundation; 2009. http://www.kff.org/medicaid/upload/7957.pdf
11. Wallace E, Hinchey T, Dimitrov BD, Bennett K, Fahey T, Smith SM. A systematic review of the probability of repeated admission score in community-dwelling adults. J Am Geriatr Soc. 2013;61(3):357–64.
12. Herr M, Ankri J. A critical review of the use of telephone tests to identify cognitive impairment in epidemiology and clinical research. J Telemed Telecare. 2013;19(1):45–54.
13. Wang L, Porter B, Maynard C, Evans G, Bryson C, Sun H, Gupta I, Lowy E, McDonell M, Frisbee K, Nielson C, Kirland F, Fihn SD. Predicting risk of hospitalization or death among patients receiving primary car in the Veterans Health Administration. Med Care. 2013;51(4):368–73.
14. Albada M, Cha SS, Takahashi PY. The elders risk assessment index, an electronic administrative database-derived frailty index, can identify risk of hip fracture in a cohort of community-dwelling adults. Mayo Clin Proc. 2012;87(7):652–8.
15. Higgins S, Chawla R, Colombo C, Snyder R, Nigam S. Medical homes and cost and utilization among high-risk patients. Am J Manag Care. 2014;20(3):e61–71.
16. Edmans JA, Gladman JRF, Havard D. Umbrella review of tools to assess risk of poor outcome in older people attending acute medical units. Medical crises in older people discussion paper series. Issue 11 2012. http://www.nottingham.ac.uk/mcop/documents/papers/issue11-mcop-issn2044-4230.pdf

17. Bixby MB, Naylor MD. The Transitional Care Model (TCM): hospital discharge screening criteria for high risk older adults. Try this: best practices in nursing care to older patients. Issue 26, 2009. http://consultgerirn.org/uploads/File/trythis/try_this_26.pdf
18. Wenger NS, Roth CP, Shekelle P, ACOVE Investigators. Introduction to assessing care of vulnerable elders-3 quality indicators measurement set. J Am Geriatr Soc. 2007;55:S247–52.
19. Grabowski DC. The cost-effectiveness of noninstitutional long-term care services: review and synthesis of the most recent evidence. Med Care Res Rev. 2006;63(1):3–28.
20. Ouwens M, Wollersheim H, Hermens R, et al. Integrated care programmes for chronically ill patients: a review of systematic reviews. Int J Qual Health Care. 2005;17(2):141–6.
21. Chiu WK, Newcomer R. A systematic review of nurse-assisted case management to improve hospital discharge transition outcomes for the elderly. Prof Case Manag. 2007;12(6):330–6.
22. Hansen LO, Young RS, Hinami K, et al. Interventions to reduce 30-day rehospitalization: a systematic review. Ann Intern Med. 2011;155(8):520–8.
23. Golden AG, Martin S, da Silva M, Roos BA. Care management and the transition of older adults from a skilled nursing facility back into the community. Care Manag J. 2011;12(2):54–9.
24. Golden AG, Tewary S, Dang S, Roos RA. Care management challenges and opportunities to reduce the rapid rehospitalization of frail community-dwelling older adults. Gerontologist. 2010;50(4):451–8.
25. Jones SS, Rudin RS, Perry T, Shekelle PG. Health information technology: an updated systematic review with a focus on meaningful use. Ann Intern Med. 2014;160:48–54.
26. Campbell KR. What are the biggest issues with EMR today? [Internet]. 2012. http://www.kevinmd.com/blog/2012/11/biggest-issue-emr-today.html. [Cited November 4, 2013].
27. Alder-Milstein J, Salzberg C, Franz C, Orav J, Newhouse JP. Effect of electronic health records on health care costs: longitudinal comparative evidence from community practice. Ann Intern Med. 2013;159(2):97–104.
28. Kaushal R. Reducing the costs of U.S. health care: the role of electronic health records. Ann Intern Med. 2013;159(2):151–2.
29. Wang CJ. Medical documentation in the electronic era. JAMA. 2012;308(20):2091–2.
30. Golden AG, Silverman MA, Wan TTH. Electronic health records: an awkward third wheel. South Med J. 2014;107(6):380.
31. Wilson SR, Cram P. Another sobering result for home telehealth- and where we might go next. Arch Intern Med. 2012;172(10):779–80.
32. Dang S, Golden AG, Cheung HS, Roos BA. Telemedicine applications in geriatrics. In: Fillit HM, Rockwood K, Woodhouse K, editors. JC Brocklehurst textbook of geriatric medicine and gerontology. 7th ed. London: Churchill Livingstone; 2010. p. 1064–9.
33. Takahashi PY, Pecina JL, Upatising B, et al. A randomized controlled trial of telemonitoring in older adults with multiple health issues to prevent hospitalizations and emergency department visits. Arch Intern Med. 2012;172(11):773–9.
34. Golden AG, Silverman MA, Mintzer MJ. Is geriatric medicine terminally ill? Ann Intern Med. 2012;156(9):654–6.
35. Cohen HJ, Feussner JR, Weinberger M, Carnes M, Hamdy RC, Hsieh F, Phibbs C, Lavori P. A controlled trial of inpatient and outpatient geriatric evaluation and management. N Engl J Med. 2002;346:905–12.
36. Ellis G, Whitehead MA, O'Neill D, Langhorne P, Robinson D. Comprehensive geriatric assessment for older adults admitted to the hospital. Cochrane Database Syst Rev. 2011;7:CD006211.
37. Fox MT, Persaud M, Maimets I, O'Brien K, Brooks D, Tregunno D, Schaa E. Effectiveness of acute geriatric unit care using actue care for elders components: a systematic review and meta-analysis. J Am Geriatr Soc. 2012;60(12):2237–45.
38. D'Souza S, Guptha S. Preventing admission of older people to hospital. BMJ. 2013;346:f30186.
39. Epstein AM, Jha AK, Orav EJ, Liebman DL, Audet AM, Zezza MA, Guterman S. Analysis of early accountable care organizations defines patient, structural, cost and quality-of-care characteristics. Health Aff. 2014;33(1):95–102.

40. Centers for Medicare and Medicaid Services. Pioneer accountable care organizations succeed in improving care, lowering costs [Internet]. 2013. www.cms.gov/newsroom. [Cited January 8, 2014].
41. Correia EW. Accountable care organizations: the proposed regulations and the prospects for success. Am J Manag Care. 2011;17(8):560–8.
42. Burns LR, Pauly MV. Accountable care organizations may have difficulty avoiding the failures of integrated delivery networks of the 1990s. Health Aff. 2012;31(11):2407–16.
43. American Academy of Family Physicians, American Academy of Pediatrics, American College of Physicians, American Osteopathic Association Joint Principles of the Patient-Centered Medical Home. 2007. http://www.acponline.org/running_practice/delivery_and_payment_models/pcmh/demonstrations/jointprinc_05_17.pdf
44. Maeng DD, Graham J, Graf TR, et al. Reducing long-term cost by transforming primary care: evidence from Geisinger's medical home mode. Am J Manag Care. 2012;18(3):149–55.
45. Friedberg MW, Schneider EC, Rosenthal MB, Volpp KG, Werner RM. Association between participation in a multipayer medical home intervention and changes in quality, utilization and costs of care. JAMA. 2014;311(8):815–25.
46. United States Congress. The Better Care Lower Cost Act of 2014. http://beta.congress.gov/bill/113th/senate-bill/1932
47. Institute of Medicine. New models of care. In: Retooling for an Aging America: building the health care workforce. Washington, DC: National Academies Press; 2008, pp. 75–122. http://www.nap.edu/catalog/12089.html
48. Meret-Haneke LA. Effects of the program of all-inclusive care for the elderly on hospital use. Gerontologist. 2011;51:774–85.
49. Golden AG, Ortiz J, Wan TT. Transitional care: looking for the right shoes to fit older adult patients? Care Manag J. 2013;14(2):78–83.
50. Department of Elder Affairs, State of Florida. Program of all-inclusive care for the elderly & statewide medicaid managed care long-term care program comparison report 2014. 2014. http://elderaffairs.state.fl.us/doea/Evaluation/PACE_Evaluation_2014.pdf
51. Counsell SR, Callahan CM, Clark DO, Tu W, Buttar AB, Stump TE, Ricketts GD. Geriatric care management for low-income seniors: a randomized controlled trial. JAMA. 2007;298(22):2623–33.
52. Counsell SR, Callahan CM, Tu W, Stump TE, Arling GW. Cost analysis of the geriatric resources for assessment and care of elders care management intervention. J Am Geriatr Soc. 2009;57(8):1420–6.
53. Medicare Payment Advisory Commission. Report to the Congress-Medicare Payment Policy. 2012. http://www.medpac.gov/documents/Mar12_EntireReport.pdf. Accessed 5 June 2012.
54. Medicare Payment Advisory Commission. Report to the Congress: Medicare payment policy. Washington, DC: MedPAC; 2009. http://www.medpac.gov/documents/Mar09_March%20report%20testimony_WM%20FINAL.pdf. Accessed 12 Aug 2012.
55. Aldridge MD, Schlesinger M, Barry CL, Morrison RS, McCorkle R, Hürzeler R, Bradley EH. National hospice survey results: for-profit status, community engagement, and survey. JAMA Intern Med. 2014;174(4):500–506.
56. Murray SA, Kendall M, Boyd K, Sheikh A. Illness trajectories and palliative care. BMJ. 2005;330(7498):1007–11.
57. Christakis NA, Lamont EB. Extent and determinants of error in doctors' prognoses in terminally ill patients: prospective cohort study. BMJ. 2000;320(7233):469–72.
58. Lamont EB, Christakis NA. Prognostic disclosures to patients with cancer near the end of life. Ann Intern Med. 2001;134(12):1096–105.
59. Edes T. Transforming VA care at the end of life [Internet]. 2010. http://council.brandeis.edu/pdfs/2010/Edes.pdf. [Cited March 10, 2014].
60. Weeks JC, Catalano PJ, Cronin A, Finkelman MD, Mack JW, Keating NL, Schraq D. Patients' expectations about effects of chemotherapy for advanced cancer. N Engl J Med. 2012;367(17):1616–25.
61. Golden AG, Roos BA, Silverman MA, Beers MH. Home and community-based Medicaid options for dependent older Floridians. J Am Geriatr Soc. 2010;58(2):371–6.

62. Grabowski DC, Cadigan RO, Miller EA, Stevenson DG, Clark M, Mor V. Supporting home and community-based care: views of long-term care specialists. Med Care Res Rev. 2010;67 (4 Suppl):82S–101.
63. Golden AG, Roos BA, Silverman MA, Wan TTH. The challenges measuring the effectiveness of a statewide Medicaid long-term care managed care program: the Florida experience. Int J Public Policy. 2012;8:43–52.
64. Mor V, Intrator O, Feng Z, Grabowski DC. The revolving door of rehospitalization from skilled nursing facilities. Health Aff. 2010;29(1):57–64.
65. Institute of Medicine. Interim report of the committee on geographic variation in health care spending and promotion of high value care: preliminary committee observations. 2013. http://books.nap.edu/openbook.php?record_id=18308. Accessed 31 Mar 2014.
66. Jencks SF, Williams MV, Coleman EA. Rehospitalizations among patients in the Medicare fee-for-service program. N Engl J Med. 2009;360(14):1418–28.
67. Centers for Medicare and Medicaid Services. Chronic conditions among Medicare Beneficiaries, Chartbook: 2012 Edition. Baltimore, MD. 2012.
68. Centers for Medicare and Medicaid Services. Community-based care transitions program. http://innovation.cms.gov/initiatives/CCTP/
69. Naylor MD, Bowles KH, McCauley KM, Maccoy MC, Maislin G, Pauly MV, Krakauer R. High-value transitional care: transition of research into practice. J Eval Clin Pract. 2013;19(5):727–33.
70. Peikes D, Zutshi A, Genevro JL, et al. Early evaluations of the medical home: building on a promising start. Am J Manag Care. 2012;18(2):105–16.
71. Ouslander JG, Bonner A, Herdon L. The Interventions to Reduce Acute Transfers (INTERACT) quality improvement program: an overview for medical directors and primary care clinicians in long term care. J Am Med Dir Assoc. 2014;15(3):162–70.
72. Ouslander JG, Lamb G, Tappen R, et al. Interventions to reduce hospitalizations from nursing homes: evaluation of the INTERACT II collaborative quality improvement project. J Am Geriatr Soc. 2011;59(4):745–53.
73. Tena-Nelson R, Santos K, Weingast E, et al. Reducing potentially preventable hospital transfers: results from a thirty nursing home collaborative. J Am Med Dir Assoc. 2012;13:651–6.
74. Gill TM, Gahbauer EA, Han L, Allore HG. Functional trajectories in older persons admitted to a nursing home with disability after an acute hospitalization. J Am Geriatr Soc. 2009;57(2):195–201.
75. Supreme Court of the United States. Opinion of the court. Olmstead v. L.C. No. 98–536. 1999. http://www.law.cornell.edu/supct/pdf/98-536P.ZO
76. Peikes D, Chen A, Schore J, Brown R. Effects of care coordination on hospitalization, quality of care, and health care expenditures among Medicare beneficiaries: 15 randomized trials. JAMA. 2009;301(6):603–18.

Chapter 11
Accountable Care Organizations: A Case Study in the Use of Care Coordination: Montefiore Medical Center

Hope Glassberg, Anne Meara, and Laurie G. Jacobs

> *America's health care system is neither healthy, caring, nor a system.*
> – Walter Cronkite

Abbreviations

ACO	Accountable Care Organization
CMHCB	Care Management for High Cost Beneficiaries
CMO	Montefiore Care Management Organization
CMS	Center for Medicare & Medicaid Services
DRG	Diagnosis Related Group
ED	Emergency Department
FFS	Fee-for-Service
HMO	Health Maintenance Organization
MIPA	Montefiore Integrated Provider Association
PCMHs	Patient Centered Medical Homes

H. Glassberg, M.P.A. • A. Meara, BSN, M.B.A.
Care Management Organization, Montefiore Medical Center,
200 Corporate Boulevard, Yonkers, NY 10701, USA
e-mail: hglassbe@montefiore.org; ameara@montefiore.org; ameara6137@aol.com

L.G. Jacobs, M.D. (✉)
Department of Medicine, Montefiore Medical Center and Albert Einstein College of Medicine, 111 East 210 Street, Bronx, NY 10467, USA
e-mail: lajacobs@montefiore.org

© Springer International Publishing Switzerland 2015
J.S. Powers (ed.), *Healthcare Changes and the Affordable Care Act*,
DOI 10.1007/978-3-319-09510-3_11

Introduction

John[1] is a 68 year-old Bronx resident with diabetes, hypertension, end-stage renal disease (ESRD), diminishing visual acuity, and poor hearing. To manage his ESRD, John undergoes dialysis over 3–4 h sessions per week at a free-standing dialysis center. Due to John's hearing impairment, he has had difficulty arranging transportation to dialysis and is frequently late or misses sessions. John sees his nephrologist at dialysis a few times monthly. Care is focused on his kidney disease, hypertension, and diabetes. He has not sought help with his hearing and visual impairments, as he is uncertain where to obtain services, is unsure who will pay for hearing aids and glasses, and does not have the time or energy to seek further medical care beyond the time spent in dialysis. As a result, he has not seen his primary care physician to discuss the other conditions, preventive care, or other specialty care. He feels socially isolated and overwhelmed at the prospect of navigating all of his healthcare needs. John has sought care in the emergency room due to uncontrolled diabetes, a respiratory infection, declining vision, and other complaints, averaging two visits and one inpatient admission per month.

John's story is not unique. Individuals across the United States increasingly suffer from multiple chronic conditions [1] and fragmented care, spread across many medical providers. An average Medicare patient sees two physicians and five specialists in a year, rising to 13 physicians a year if they have a chronic disease [2]. This level of fragmentation is compounded by social burdens, such as lack of social supports or a caregiver, unstable housing, domestic violence, and poverty. The implications of fragmentation are significant: patients may obtain duplicative care, receive discordant diagnoses or medications, or use emergency departments as one-stop-shop sources of services [3, 4], thereby missing out on continuity of care for chronic conditions or preventive care.

Accountable care organization (ACO) models described in the prior chapter, as well as other care coordination models like Patient Centered Medical Homes (PCMHs), seek to break this pattern. These models presume that if delivery systems help patients navigate and manage their conditions across healthcare settings, they will get the right care, in the right place, at the right time.

Care coordination, broadly speaking, is defined by the Agency for Healthcare Research and Quality as "deliberately organizing patient care activities and sharing information among all of the participants concerned with a patient's care to achieve safer and more effective care" [5]. This chapter describes how Montefiore Medical Center has implemented care coordination efforts within the context of ACO and ACO-like programs.

---

[1] Composite based upon multiple cases.

Montefiore Medical Center: Transforming Managed Care into Care Management

Montefiore Medical Center is an urban academic medical center based in the Bronx, and lower Westchester County, New York, which serves over one million individuals annually. Montefiore's integrated delivery system spans five general and one children's hospital, over 20 community-based primary care centers, seven mobile healthcare units, four emergency departments, three major specialty care centers, a home care agency, and other specialty programs.

Montefiore, initially established in 1884 to serve individuals with chronic disease, has a mission to serve vulnerable, underserved populations within its community [6]. In 1950, Montefiore created the nation's first Hospital Department of Social Medicine, followed by a residency program in social medicine and pediatrics, designed to train future healthcare providers to deploy clinical expertise to communities with poor access and a high intensity of social and health problems [6, 7].

Since that time, Montefiore has expanded its service delivery via a wide range of hospital and community-based programs to provide high quality medical care and social supports to a rapidly expanding and increasingly diverse community. The history of some of these activities is described below, along with specific discussion of Montefiore's activities in the context of the Pioneer ACO program.[2]

Care Coordination at Montefiore

Early on, Montefiore sought to promote continuity of care for its patient population by developing a robust network of providers beyond the hospital walls. In the 1960s, Montefiore was deeply involved in the establishment of an early federally designated neighborhood health center, the Dr. Martin Luther King Health Center, with an explicit mission to deliver "social rehabilitation of a whole neighborhood, as a way to break the vicious cycle of poverty" [8, 9].

Recognizing a tremendous ongoing need for such services, Montefiore continued to expand its network of primary care centers in the Bronx, including some federally qualified health centers, as well as other practices. Montefiore also opened the first Home Care Program and added a long-term care facility to its expanding list of services. By the early 2000s, Montefiore was running over two dozen primary care practices along with targeted primary care services located in schools, homeless shelters, and other settings [6].

Concurrent with efforts to expand the population served and the continuum of health care services, Montefiore undertook partnerships with health plans to alter

---

[2] Montefiore Medical Center is operating New York's only Pioneer Accountable Care Organization (ACO). The Pioneer ACO is a federal demonstration to promote high quality coordinated care for Medicare FFS beneficiaries; the model is described at length in the previous chapter.

the framework for payments in order to incentivize a holistic model of patient care. In the 1980s, Montefiore executed an agreement with Maxicare, a Los Angeles based Health Maintenance Organization (HMO), to begin organizing its providers to collaborate with U.S. Healthcare, later acquired by Aetna.

Through this partnership and mirroring a model Maxicare pioneered in California, Montefiore participated in a group of local providers that assumed responsibility for managing hospital services and costs. Another group of providers situated within Montefiore's outpatient sites took responsibility for outpatient services. Under these arrangements, the two groups provided determinations of medical necessity (also known as utilization management [10]) on behalf of U.S. Healthcare and monitored penalties for non-timely submissions of claims for patients receiving care within and outside of the Montefiore system.

Other changes in hospital reimbursement had an impact upon Montefiore's relationships with health plans. In the 1970s and 1980s, a number of states, including New York, sought to reduce dramatic increases in hospital spending by transferring control of payment rate setting to state institutions [11]. In New York, this system evolved to one where Medicare and Medicaid paid the same rate to hospitals for given Diagnosis Related Groups (DRGs) [12], while commercial payment rates were pegged to 113 % of rates paid by non-profit insurer Blue Cross [11]. This practice eventually drew to a close in the mid-1990s with the New York Health Reform Act of 1996, which eliminated the fixed DRG payment system and required hospitals to negotiate directly with health plans to establish payment rates [13].

The changing reimbursement environment, the growing number of managed care plans nationally, and the demise of Maxicare in the New York market [14], all created a catalyst for further innovation within the Montefiore system. Building upon Montefiore's longstanding commitment to community-based care across the continuum and early population management activities, Montefiore consolidated the two groups that had managed hospital and outpatient costs into a single integrated practice association, the Montefiore Integrated Provider Association (MIPA), in the mid-1990s.

The purpose of the MIPA was to collectively act as a liaison to health plans and, wherever possible, advance arrangements through which health plans would delegate utilization management responsibility to Montefiore. The idea of such delegation, as had been the case in earlier years with Maxicare, was that staff with close ties to the delivery system would be optimally positioned to make decisions about medically necessary services. Under such arrangements, plans would share a percentage of premium dollars to Montefiore to take on this responsibility.

The Montefiore Care Management Organization (CMO) was established in parallel to the IPA as a separate wholly-owned subsidiary, tasked with training and deploying staff to provide utilization management. Montefiore also created University Behavioral Associations to assume expertise in managing behavioral health needs. The CMO was structured as a separate entity so that there was meaningful separation between financial negotiations and clinical determinations. Of note, this provider-driven care management approach far pre-dated accountable care organization models (Fig. 11.1).

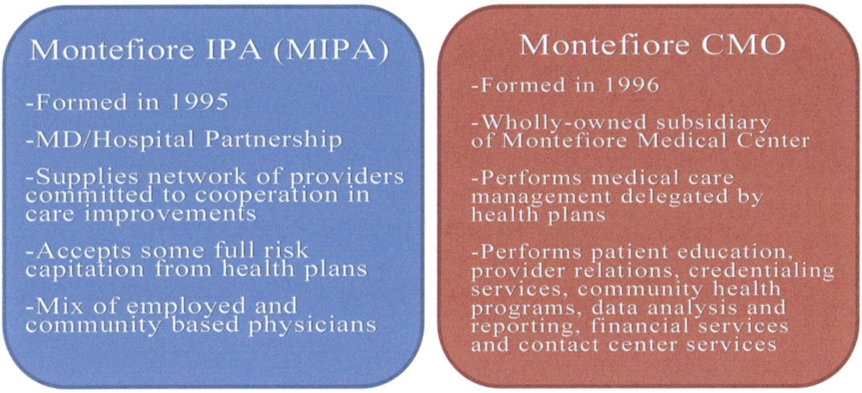

Montefiore IPA (MIPA)
- Formed in 1995
- MD/Hospital Partnership
- Supplies network of providers committed to cooperation in care improvements
- Accepts some full risk capitation from health plans
- Mix of employed and community based physicians

Montefiore CMO
- Formed in 1996
- Wholly-owned subsidiary of Montefiore Medical Center
- Performs medical care management delegated by health plans
- Performs patient education, provider relations, credentialing services, community health programs, data analysis and reporting, financial services and contact center services

Fig. 11.1 Montefiore IPA versus the CMO

In addition to reimbursement changes, Montefiore's patients molded the eventual structure of its approach to population management. The Bronx is the poorest urban county in the nation, with more than a quarter of the population living below the poverty line [15]. The acute and chronic disease burden within the Bronx is higher than elsewhere in New York City and the nation. The county posts the highest rates of diabetes, asthma, and chronic obstructive pulmonary disease hospitalizations in New York City [16] and in the South Bronx, nearly a quarter of residents do not have a doctor they visit regularly [17].

Given this environment, the CMO's scope of activities expanded beyond determinations of medical necessity to a broader "care guidance" approach that today targets not simply medical conditions, but the underlying social determinants of health. This expansion of scope was magnified in 2000, when Montefiore assumed ownership of a number of outpatient sites across the region that had previously been owned by the Health Insurance Plan of New York (HIP), and care management responsibility for tens of thousands of patients who sought medical care at those sites. Additionally, over time, the care management approach evolved as both health plan payers become more acquainted with the model and Montefiore formalized and broadened its strategies for managing care for larger populations.

Currently, the Montefiore IPA and CMO manage care for more than 200,000 beneficiaries (Fig. 11.2). The following section describes the CMO's care management approach, known as the care guidance program, in greater detail.

Component Parts of the Montefiore Care Guidance Program

Over time, Montefiore has refined its process for managing care for large populations and identifying where to focus resources.

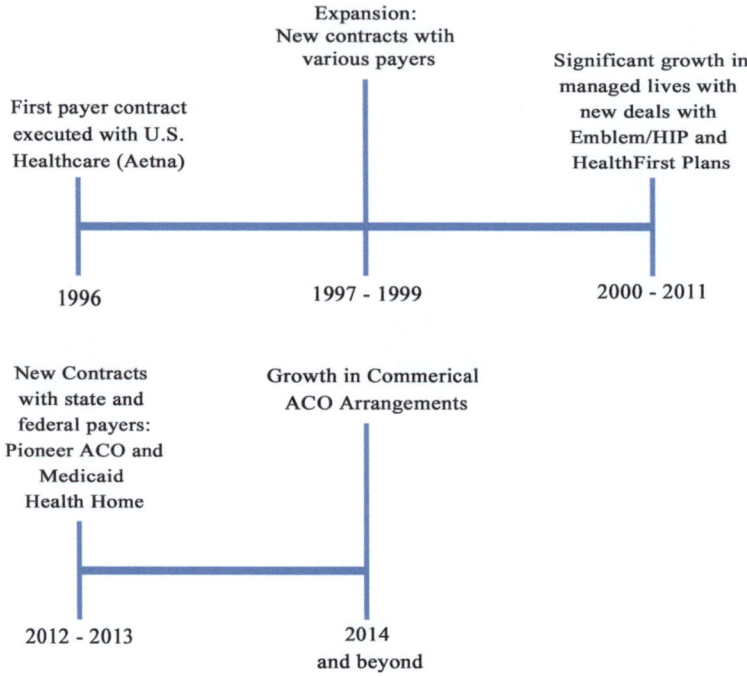

Fig. 11.2 Montefiore IPA and CMO population management timeline

Staff

When the Montefiore CMO began operations, a small group of registered nurses, physicians, and administrative staff carried out clinical activities. Over time, the CMO has expanded its scope of care management operations requiring the addition of other professional staff, including licensed practical nurses, social workers, nurse practitioners, pharmacists, dieticians, health educators and others, to facilitate engagement with patients and improve the quality and accessibility of their care. Non-clinical personnel are often best suited to engage with patients beyond the services provided by physicians and registered nurses, particularly if social issues, such as housing, impede compliance with medical management.

The CMO also works intimately with physician leaders and providers assisting them to help their patients obtain the care that they require. The Montefiore CMO employs a medical director and a team of associate medical directors to assist in overseeing utilization management activities, provide input into clinical programs, and, in some cases, manage particularly challenging patients. This team also helps in the development of outpatient PCMH activities in Montefiore network practices. Finally, the CMO medical directors serve as important peer liaisons to other physicians in the community and hospital, providing education about the care management approach and potential areas for collaboration.

CMO Structure

The Montefiore CMO operates in a primarily telephonic, centralized manner, as many patients see multiple providers across a variety of sites and needs arise outside of the doctor's office. Having a flexible, centralized resource allows clinical staff to often reach patients before an emergency situation arises and to more easily coordinate transitions of care across settings. Every day, hundreds of care management staff within the Montefiore CMO interact with patients, their providers, and care givers through the phone to develop, implement, and monitor care management interventions.

The Montefiore Care Management organization is entirely integrated with the delivery system, with some staff and resources physically situated within doctor's offices or hospitals, or deployed within the community. In Montefiore's experience, the hybrid centralized and field-based approach maximizes the ability to meet patients where they are most comfortable.

Other elements of the care management approach at Montefiore include Emergency Department (ED) navigators, who identify patients under management who seek care in the ED. The navigators alert relevant CMO staff, and, with input from those staff along with other ED personnel, devise a reasonable discharge plan and services. Additionally, Montefiore CMO certified diabetes educators work in outpatient practices to coach patients on dietary choices and other factors that impact their disease. Finally, Montefiore manages a house calls program through which providers deliver care at home for patients who are unable to travel to appointments.

Care Guidance Approach

The care guidance approach consists of standard component parts, described below. Montefiore has also developed a sophisticated information technology platform to help support these activities (Fig. 11.3):

- **Identification of Eligibility:** Montefiore has an in-house data analytics process to identify individuals who may require targeted interventions to address their

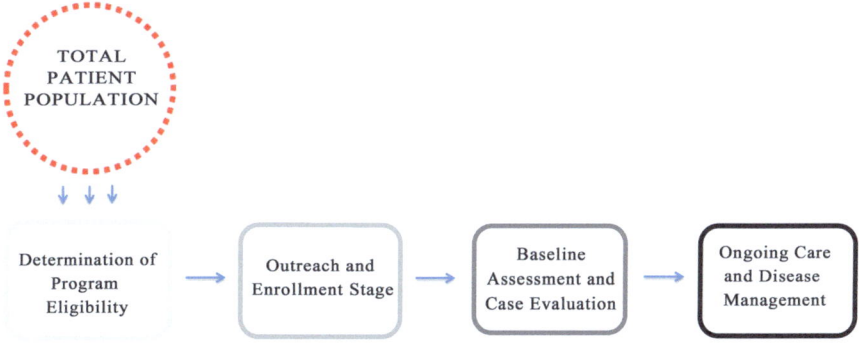

Fig. 11.3 Montefiore care guidance approach

health and social needs, based upon claims and utilization patterns; the CMO also accepts referrals from providers within the delivery system. In order to be eligible, individuals must be enrolled in a health plan with which Montefiore has a relationship or be involved in a demonstration program (the Pioneer ACO, for example) in which Montefiore participates.

- **Outreach and Enrollment:** During this stage, Montefiore CMO staff reaches out to all identified individuals and refer those who are willing to a team for a more detailed baseline assessment. Participation is entirely voluntary and free to the patient.
- **Baseline Assessment and Evaluation:** For those who are willing, the CMO staff conduct a comprehensive medical and psychosocial assessment to evaluate the full spectrum of individuals' needs. This assessment often requires multiple conversations, not simply with patients, but with care givers, and other providers. At the close of the baseline assessment and evaluation, CMO staff develop a care plan consisting of a problem list of areas requiring attention and proposed interventions to address these issues.
- **Ongoing Management:** Depending on the results of the baseline assessment and evaluation, patients may be connected to various programs:
  - *Disease Management:* the CMO operates programs to address diabetes, end-stage-renal disease, chronic kidney disease, heart failure, asthma, COPD, behavioral care, and is planning other initiatives.
  - *Intensive Case Management*: In certain cases involving individuals with very serious illness, the CMO will also connect them to interdisciplinary care teams that provide more intensive case management.
  - *Other Supports:* The CMO has a number of other specialized programs to support patients, such as a palliative care program, a pharmacy management program, and a "housing at risk" program for individuals who have no or unstable housing arrangements.

Applying Care Guidance in a Fee-For-Service (FFS) Context: The Pioneer ACO

To start, Montefiore applied its care guidance approach to populations of patients enrolled in Medicare, Medicaid, and commercial managed care plans. Eventually, Montefiore began taking responsibility for managing fee-for-service (FFS) populations in the Medicare program.

Unlike individuals who enroll in managed care plans, Medicare FFS populations do not have to choose a primary care provider and have only minimal restrictions on the network of providers whom they can see. Several organizations, including the Medicare Payment Advisory Commission, have noted that the FFS reimbursement system frequently results in poorly coordinated care: duplicative medical testing, polypharmacy, limited communication among providers, compromised care transitions, and avoidable emergency department use [18].

These features make care coordination all the more important in a FFS context. Montefiore first began coordinating care for Medicare FFS beneficiaries through the

Center for Medicare & Medicaid Services' (CMS) Care Management for High Cost Beneficiaries (CMHCB) demonstration program, which was undertaken at six organizations nationally, including Montefiore, in 2005.

Under the CMHCB, participating organizations were paid a monthly fee to manage and coordinate care for defined populations of high cost Medicare FFS beneficiaries with chronic conditions. Organizations could also access further dollars if they reduced costs associated with these beneficiary populations by 5 %, beyond the costs of the care management fee. At the outset of this demonstration, the CMO formalized its care guidance approach, establishing a standard baseline/assessment process and a supporting information technology (IT) infrastructure.

In 2012, Montefiore was chosen as 1 of 32 organizations nationally to participate in a new federal demonstration called the Pioneer ACO initiative to serve Medicare FFS beneficiaries (see prior chapter for detailed discussion). Unlike CMHCB, the Pioneer ACO program encompasses a broader population of Medicare FFS beneficiaries beyond those incurring high costs, and has different financial parameters.

Montefiore brought its experience in the CMHCB demo and years of population management to bear in this more recent FFS demonstration. From the CMO's vantage point, the Pioneer ACO has represented another variation on the theme of its existing population management activities. In other words, because FFS is simply a reimbursement type rather than a clinical classification, ACO patients receive the same care guidance supports that any other patients served by the CMO receive.

The Pioneer ACO has, however, enabled the CMO to access claims information about the Medicare FFS population it serves, enabling better insights into utilization and activities outside of the Montefiore system and therefore more comprehensive care management. The ACO initiative has also spurred on important new information exchange and further program development, including regular meetings of clinical leaders within the Montefiore system, community-based providers, and hospital administrators, to address quality improvement, technical challenges, and other implementation issues.

Montefiore is currently in the third year of the Pioneer ACO demonstration and early results are very promising. Montefiore was the top financial performer in the program in the first year of the demonstration and achieved notable outcomes among the ACO population, including a 10 % reduction in inpatient admissions and a 45 % reduction in inpatient admissions for patients with diabetes.[3]

Conclusion

John, the Bronx resident facing diabetes, hypertension, ESRD, speech and hearing impairments, was eventually connected to the Montefiore CMO for evaluation and was enrolled in one of the CMO's intensive case management programs known as Chronic Care Management.

---

[3] Based upon internal analysis

Through this program, John was connected with a CMO care manager who helped arrange transportation to dialysis appointments, assisted him in obtaining a hearing evaluation and hearing aids, and scheduled an eye examination which resulted in a new eyeglass prescription. The care manager has provided nursing support and organized physician home visits to help John manage his other medical conditions and ensure that he receives preventive care such as vaccinations. As a result, John's utilization of the emergency room and hospital has dramatically dropped off; he has been admitted to the hospital once in the past 6 months and had one additional ED emergency room visit during this timeframe, compared to nearly monthly visits previously.

The care manager also worked with the New York City Parks Department to identify a low-cost gym membership for John so that he could focus on strength training, which may now enable him to be eligible for kidney transplantation. As his health has stabilized, his outlook on life has improved and he has resumed social contact with friends from his church.

John's story illustrates how care management interventions that extend beyond episodic interactions in doctor's offices or emergency rooms and address the social determinants of health can yield meaningful results.

References

1. Bodenheimer T, Chen E, Bennett H. Confronting the growing burden of chronic disease: can the U.S. health care workforce do the job? Health Aff. 2009;28(1):64–74. http://content.healthaffairs.org/content/28/1/64.full. Accessed 28 Mar 2014.
2. Elhauge E. The fragmentation of U.S. healthcare. New York: Oxford University Press; 2010. http://www.law.harvard.edu/faculty/elhauge/pdf/Elhauge%20The%20Fragmentation%20of%20US%20Health%20Care%20-%20Introductory%20Chpt.pdf. Accessed 29 Mar 2014.
3. Rivas A. Americans explain why they prefer 'one-stop-shop' ERs instead of doctors' offices when they fall ill. Medical Daily. 9 July 2013. http://www.medicaldaily.com/poor-americans-explain-why-they-prefer-one-stop-shop-ers-instead-doctors-offices-when-they-fall-ill. Accessed 30 Mar 2014.
4. Uscher-Pines L, Pines J, Kellerman A, Gillen E, Mehotra A. Emergency department visits for nonurgent conditions: systematic literature review. Am J Manag Care. 2013;19(1):47–59. http://www.ajmc.com/publications/issue/2013/2013-1-vol19-n1/Emergency-Department-Visits-for-Nonurgent-Conditions-Systematic-Literature-Review/#sthash.zsM6JVgK.dpuf. Accessed 30 Mar 2014.
5. Agency for Healthcare Research and Quality. Care coordination. http://www.ahrq.gov/professionals/prevention-chronic-care/improve/coordination/index.html. Accessed 28 Mar 2014.
6. Foreman S. Montefiore Medical Center in the Bronx, New York: improving health in an urban community. Acad Med. 2004;79:1154–61. http://www.ilr.cornell.edu/healthcare/upload/Montefiore-Spencer-Foreman.pdf. Accessed 29 Mar 2014.
7. Montefiore Medical Center. Professional training programs. http://www.montefiore.org/family-social-medicine-professional-training-programs. Accessed 29 Mar 2014.
8. Dr. Martin Luther King, Jr. Health Center. Our programs and services. http://www.mlkhealthcenter.com/About%20Us.html. Accessed 28 Mar 2014.
9. Montefiore Medical Center. History and milestones. http://www.montefiore.org/about-history-and-milestones. Accessed 30 Mar 2014.

10. Stricker P. The role of utilization management in case management. Case Management Society of America. http://www.cmsa.org/Individual/NewsEvents/HealthTechnologyArticles/tabid/649/Default.aspx. Accessed 28 Mar 2014.
11. Atkinson G. State hospital rate setting revisited. 2009. http://www.commonwealthfund.org/Publications/Issue-Briefs/2009/Oct/State-Hospital-Rate-Setting-Revisited.aspx. Accessed 28 Mar 2014.
12. Centers for Medicare and Medicaid Services. Acute hospital inpatient prospective payment system fact sheet. 2013. http://www.cms.gov/Outreach-and-Education/Medicare-Learning-Network-MLN/MLNProducts/downloads/AcutePaymtSysfctsht.pdf. Accessed 28 Mar 2014.
13. Robert Wood Johnson Foundation. Study of the effects of the New York Health Care Reform Act of 1996 on health service access and efficiency. http://www.rwjf.org/en/grants/grant-records/1997/10/study-of-the-effects-of-the-new-york-health-care-reform-act-of-1.html. Accessed 28 Mar 2014.
14. Freudenheim M. Business and health; Maxicare's plan to cut losses. The New York Times. 3 May 1988. http://www.nytimes.com/1988/05/03/business/business-and-health-maxicare-s-plan-to-cut-losses.html. Accessed 30 Mar 2014.
15. Meminger D. Report cites Bronx as poorest urban county. NY1. 2009. http://www.ny1.com/content/news/106559/report-cites-bronx-as-poorest-urban-county/. Accessed 28 Mar 2014.
16. New York City Department of Health and Mental Hygiene. Epiquery: NYC interactive health data system – community health survey 2010. Last updated: 2/2013. http://nyc.gov/health/epiquery
17. New York City Department of Health and Mental Hygiene. Community health profile: Southeast Bronx. http://www.nyc.gov/html/doh/downloads/pdf/data/2006chp-104.pdf. Accessed 30 Mar 2014.
18. Medicare Payment Advisory Commission. Report to the Congress. 2012, chap. 2. http://www.google.com/url?sa=t&rct=j&q=&esrc=s&source=web&cd=1&cad=rja&uact=8&ved=0CCwQFjAA&url=http%3A%2F%2Fwww.medpac.gov%2Fchapters%2FJun12_Ch02.pdf&ei=SykbU-CDOuPv0wHinYGYAg&usg=AFQjCNGq-tuB-TZj5HHGrRWe7SYZMrH04w&sig2=bLymdskHpLU7aUV-eCuJgw&bvm=bv.62578216,d.dmQ. Accessed 29 Mar 2014.

Chapter 12
University of Michigan Case Study: The Physician Group Practice Demonstration

Caroline S. Blaum, Brent C. Williams, and David A. Spahlinger

Abbreviations

BCBSM	Blue Cross Blue Shield of Michigan
CCMP	Complex Care Management Program
CMMI	Centers for Medicaid and Medicare Innovation
EMR	Electronic Medical Record
HCC	Heirarchical Claims Categories
M*STARR	Michigan-State Action on Avoidable Rehospitalizations
MSSP	Medicare Shared Savings Program
NCQA	National Committee for Quality Assurance
PCMH	Patient Centered Medical Home
PGPD	Physician Group Practice Demonstration
QMP	Quality Management Program
UMHS	University of Michigan Healthcare System

C.S. Blaum, M.D., M.S. (✉)
Department of Medicine, Division of Geriatric Medicine and Palliative Care,
NYU School of Medicine, NYU Langone Medical Center, 550 First Ave, BCD612,
New York, NY 10016, USA
e-mail: Caroline.Blaum@nyumc.org

B.C. Williams, M.D., MPH
Internal Medicine, University of Michigan, 2800 Plymouth Road,
North Campus Research Complex, Building 16, Room 447E, Ann Arbor, MI 48109, USA
e-mail: bwilliam@umich.edu

D.A. Spahlinger, M.D.
Internal Medicine, University of Michigan, 1301 Catherine Street, 4114 Med Sci I,
Ann Arbor, MI 48109-5624, USA
e-mail: dspahlin@umich.edu

© Springer International Publishing Switzerland 2015
J.S. Powers (ed.), *Healthcare Changes and the Affordable Care Act*,
DOI 10.1007/978-3-319-09510-3_12

Introduction

A fundamental question in health policy is how the newly forming Accountable Care Organizations (ACO) will achieve high quality and efficient care for patients and populations. In Medicare there are nearly 300 Accountable Care Organizations in two major programs: the Pioneer Demonstration, which involves more financial risk for the ACO, and the Medicare Shared Savings Program, which has less risk [1]. These ACO's have been operating for about 2 years and information is beginning to be released about their performance. However, there are already several years of information from an important precursor to Medicare ACO's – the Physician Group Practice Demonstration (PGPD) [2]. The University of Michigan (UM) was one of ten large physician organizations that participated in the PGPD from 2005 to 2010. Two groups, including the UM, were very successful and achieved shared savings and quality targets for all 5 years of the Demonstration. Seven of the groups eventually earned shared savings (two groups for 1 year only, two groups for 2 years, one group for 3 years and two groups for all 5 years) reaching about $100 million in savings for Medicare over the 5 years, and $80 million in aggregate shared savings distributed among successful groups [2]. The University of Michigan saved Medicare about $22 million and received $17.6 million in shared savings over the 5 years of the PGPD. All groups had high quality, as measured by ambulatory quality measures similar to current PQRS (Physician Quality Reporting System) [3, 4] measures of physician clinical performance in major chronic diseases (diabetes, heart failure, CAD) and in preventative care.

Reviews and analysis of the PGPD have appeared in the literature over the past few years, and analyses are available on the CMS website [2]. Although many policy makers and researchers do not consider the PGPD a success [5, 6], it was one of the prototypes and inspirations for the current ACO demonstrations and programs. Those who consider it a qualified success [7–9] generally cite structural and organizational characteristics of the PGPD groups, their electronic medical record (EMR), risk adjustment, and care coordination infrastructure. Although these characteristics are important, it is not possible for policy makers to understand this complex sociomedical quasi-experiment at the level of the individual healthcare system by reviewing claims and interviewing participants. This chapter explores the University of Michigan's characteristics and care processes that contributed to its financial success within the particular structural and financial model of the PGPD.

Brief Overview of the PGPD

The structure of the PGPD included retrospective patient assignment to each participating physician group based on the plurality of outpatient E&M costs. Retrospective assignment means that patients were assigned to the University of Michigan at the end of each performance year depending upon the pleurality of theirs costs, and therefore, during the performance year, UMHS did not know if a particular patient would eventually be assigned. The assignment was based on the Tax ID number of the physicians (TIN), and the University of Michigan Healthcare System (UMHS), as a large, integrated healthcare system, has one TIN for its providers. The PGPD participants were responsible for all Medicare costs incurred by their assigned patients (except for Medicare D) no matter where the care was received. Because the PGPD, like current ACO's, was part of fee for service Medicare, patients could receive care from the PGPD participating group practice, or anywhere else. Medicare D was excluded because those costs were covered by Medicare through the Medicare D program and not through the PGPD [4].

As with current ACO's, the financial goal was to "bend the curve" or decrease Medicare growth compared to the Medicare growth of the local market area. The financial model measured risk adjusted growth compared to the local area risk adjusted growth, referenced to an unchanging baseline year. Shared savings were 80 % of savings beyond a 2 % corridor. This risk corridor is analogous to a confidence interval in statistics and meant that PGPD participants had to save at least 2 % before savings were available to share. (For example, if a PGPD participant saved 2.1 %, they only shared in 0.1 % of the savings.) Risk adjustment was done based on customized, claims based algorithm that accounted for burden of disease called hierarchical claims categories (HCC's) [10].

In order to receive shared savings, assuming the participating physician group had decreased Medicare growth and was eligible, the physician group practice had to achieve quality targets on 32 ambulatory quality measures which were measures for chronic disease and prevention similar to current Medicare Physician Quality Reporting System [11] measures. Seven of these were measured by claims and 25 were done by chart review of a sample of beneficiaries, similar to HEDIS methodology. Just about all these structural characteristics were changed for both the Pioneer ACO Demonstration Program and the Medicare Shared Savings Program (MSSP).

Characteristics Associated with UMHS's Success in the PGPD

A true understanding of which healthcare system characteristics led to UM's success in the PGPD would require analyzing data from the local market area comparison group (south eastern and south central Michigan), and some of the published literature does make use of these data [12, 13]. However, some insight is given by the fact that the UMHS has several characteristics widely considered important for success in efficient care of Medicare patients. These characteristics include: integrated structure with coordinated governance and employed physicians; system-wide electronic medical record (EMR); managed care/risk experience including capacity for administrative data analysis; and care coordination infrastructure across the care continuum.

Integrated Structure and Electronic Medical Record (EMR)

The University of Michigan Medical School and Hospital and Health System is part of the University of Michigan (UM) [14]. UM is a constitutional entity of the State of Michigan and final authority resides with the Board of Regents elected by the voters of the State of Michigan. The Medical School and Hospital and Health Clinics are integrated into the University of Michigan Health System (UMHS). UMHS is led by an Executive Vice President of Medical Affairs, to whom the CEO of the Hospital and Health Clinics and the Dean of the Medical School report, and who in turn reports to the President of the University of Michigan. Table 12.1 shows UMHS characteristics. All physicians are salaried faculty of the Medical School, and salaries are generally determined by a complex performance review related to academic (research, teaching) and clinical (mainly productivity and compliance with clinical quality measures) metrics. The mix of academic and clinical activities varies widely among faculty physicians. The Faculty Group Practice is the structure that organizes and manages the clinical activities of the UM Medical School faculty, and is a large multispecialty group practice. UMHS also includes a home health care agency and a DME/infusion/orthotics group.

Table 12.1 University of Michigan health system characteristics (current)

***Integrated* Academic healthcare system, within a major public research university**	
Total available/staffed beds: **960**	
Inpatient discharges (excl. newborns): 45,429	
Clinic visits per year (all sites excluding ER): 1,875,186	
Emergency/urgent care visits: 97,546	
U-M Medical school	
Enrollment: 652 m	
NIH fiscal year 2008 awards: $284.4 million (11th highest among U.S. medical schools)	
Faculty and staff	
U-M health system total: 21,311	
Nurses: 3,874	
Faculty: 2516	
114 primary care FTE	
House officers: 1,239	
Health system	
3 hospitals	
48 health centers	
23 primary care practices	
Home care agency	
Number of Medicare patients seen/year: varies by year, usually about 40,000	
Number of Medicare patients attributed to PGP Demo in 2005–2010: varied by year, usually about 19,000/year	
$2.7 billion patient care revenues	

During the PGPD, UMHS had a uniform, patient-centered, web-based EMR in the hospital, ambulatory clinical areas, home health and DME. This EMR supported provider notes, as well as other clinical and administrative (scheduling, billing) data. For most of the PGPD, chronic disease registries were programmed into the EMR and used to support ambulatory quality measurement and performance improvement (see below). During the last years of the PGPD, the EMR supported computerized order entry and ePrescribing. About 2 years after the PGPD ended, UMHS migrated to the Epic EMR system.

Experience with Managed Care and Provider Risk

UMHS has substantial experience with managed care and provider risk. From 1985 to 2006 UMHS owned and operated MCARE, a full service, wholly owned Managed Care Organization eventually covering over 200,000 lives in Southeast and South Central Michigan. MCARE operated traditional HMO, PPO, and Point of Service products for regional employers, as well as a Qualified Health Plan for Medicaid in Michigan. From 1997 to 2002 MCARE included a Medicare risk plan (Medicare Plus Choice). UMHS providers took full risk for their assigned populations, including commercial (HMO, PPO, POS), Medicaid, and Medicare for most of MCARE's existence. MCARE was financially sound at the time it was sold to Blue Cross Blue Shield of Michigan (BCBSM) in 2006. Many of the UMHS physician and administrative leaders, and skilled claims and administrative data analysts who were involved in MCARE went on to lead population-based clinical transformation efforts, including the PGPD, and continue to be involved to this day with several similar clinical redesign efforts in which the UMHS is involved.

UMHS's experience with population management during the 1990s–2000s also included innovative provider-based health-care plans UMHS operated for salaried employees, dependents and retirees of the Ford Motor Company (Partnership Health) and GM (Active Health). These were population-based, company funded products in which the care delivery model and benefit structure were jointly designed by the UMHS and employers to improve care coordination and align incentives. These plans featured many elements now included in many ACO and Patient – Centered Medical Home (PCMH) care delivery models as well as other innovative features (member selection of a coordinating physician, personalized care plans that could be used to change plan benefits, care coordination through nurse navigators, and disease management programs) [15]. Although these plans were terminated during the downturn in the auto industry, evaluation at the time demonstrated savings and improved clinical quality, particularly for patients with chronic diseases.

The University of Michigan is self-insured and bears full risk for about 80,000 employees, dependents, and retirees who receive the vast majority of their care through UMHS. UMHS also accepts risk for approximately 10,000 Medicaid managed care patients. In addition to this insurance risk, UMHS has multiple performance-based payment arrangements for both hospital and professional payments. The state of Michigan has a dominant insurer, Blue Cross and Blue Shield of Michigan (BCBSM) that also has a managed care component, Blue Care Network. Through BCBSM, which insured many of its commercial patients, UMHS participated in performance-based payment programs for the hospital, and for physician performance in the management of chronic disease for several years before and during the PGPD. The BCBSM performance-based payment program helps to support UMHS's chronic disease registry development and some chronic disease quality improvement activities. Eventually, BCBSM incentivized development of a Patient Centered Medical Home (PCMH) model for commercial patients. As the primary care clinics became certified as PCMH's for commercial patients, Medicare and Medicaid patients were also included. The PCMH was developing during the last year of the PGPD. Because of this experience UMHS also participates in a Center for Medicaid and Medicare Innovation Demonstration that involved PCMH development for Medicare and Medicaid patients, the all-payer Advanced Primary Care Demonstration, which began in late 2011.

Clinical Redesign and Models of Care

The integrated structure of the UMHS, its system-wide EMR, and its experience with managed care and both insurance and performance risk were major factors when UMHS decided to participate in the PGPD in 2005. The healthcare system leadership believed then (and still does) that a new business model is coming and UMHS, as an Academic Medical Center, needs to learn how to operate in this emerging business environment. The strategy adopted to improve efficiency and quality of care for Medicare beneficiaries at UMHS involved clinical redesign and models of care and had three key elements: (1) avoid unnecessary re-hospitalizations: (2) coordinate care of high risk, high cost Medicare beneficiaries, including the frail elderly and or dual eligible (enrolled in both Medicaid and Medicare) patients; and (3) coordinate with care delivery models and innovations that were already in place at UMHS, many "left over" from managed care experiences.

This strategy led to the development or enhancement of clinical programs related to transitional care, including a large sub-acute care service in community nursing homes [16], care management of dual eligible patients and frail elders, and a renewed focus on and coordination among existing clinical programs that had grown up during the 1990s when managed care was growing. In addition, in order to meet the quality requirements of the PGPD, a clinical quality improvement program based on physician feed-back and chronic disease registries was able to make use of the infrastructure that was being developed for commercial patients and to enhance this infrastructure for Medicare beneficiaries. Table 12.2 lists these programs and their key characteristics; these programs are described in more detail in the following sections. When the PGPD ended, UMHS participated in the Transition Demonstration from 1/1/2011 to 12/31/2011 (which tests several design features of the Pioneer ACO and MSSP); the Pioneer ACO Demonstration from 1/1/2012 to

Table 12.2 Proportion of attributed patients affected by the major clinical care and quality improvement interventions at UMHS during Physician Group Practice Demonstration: Performance Year 5 example

Intervention	Year started	% of attributed patients in year 5 experiencing the intervention	Description
Post-acute call-back program	2005–	25 %	Ensure PCP follow-up and home care services as needed, understanding and access to medications
Complex care coordination program	2005–	1 %	Care coordination for dual eligible and uninsured patients with combined mental health and medical conditions
Geriatrics clinical programs	2005–	10 %	Multidisciplinary primary care, care coordination, and palliative care services
Sub-acute geriatrics faculty service	2006–	2.5 %	Subacute care services and transition care coordination among subacute, hospital, and primary care settings
PGIP quality programs with chronic disease registries	2006–	44 %	Care coordination and clinical management for patients with dominant diseases such as cancer, congestive heart failure, and diabetes
Michigan Medical Home (primary care)	2009–	Varies by year, usually about 50 %	Specific features of PCP practices to facilitate access, coordination, communication, disease self-management in primary care practices

12/31/2012, and changed to the CMS MSSP program on 1/1/2013 when it partnered with several large physician groups in Southern Michigan. In addition, since 2012 UMHS has participated in the Michigan Primary Care Transformation (MiPCT) project, a 3-year, multi-payer, project implemented in eight states aimed at reforming primary care payment models and expanding the capabilities of patient-centered medical homes (PCMH).

Clinical Models to Avoid Unnecessary Re-Hospitalizations

Transitional Care Programs

The University of Michigan Faculty Group Practice implemented a transitional care and complex care management program shortly after beginning participation in the PGPD in 2005 [17]. These related programs use the same team, which initially consisted of 4.5 nurses, 2 social workers, and 2 patient care advocates, supported by a physician medical director (the complex care management program is described below). The centerpiece of both is a post-acute care call-back program to address the poor coordination between the acute and ambulatory care settings, and to identify complex patients being discharged from the hospital or Emergency Department (ED).

Additional transitional care programs were developed over the 5 years of the PGPD and eventually included: acute-care discharge process redesign; transitional care clinics in geriatrics and cardiology; a sub-acute service in local high volume skilled nursing (e.g. sub-acute care) facilities; and finally implementation of transitional care coordination in all U-M primary care clinics as the PCMH program was rolled out and the PGPD was ending.

The post-acute callback program focused on Medicare patients discharged from the hospital or the ED. Since mid-2005 this program has called about up to 15,000 patients per year discharged from the UM hospital or ED within 24 h of discharge during the week; Friday and weekend discharges are called on Monday. The post-acute call-back program consists of a team of nurses, nurse assistants and social workers, as described above, supported by a physician medical director with direct access to a consultant pharmacist and a home care service provider. The team focuses on complex Medicaid, Medicare, dual-eligible and uninsured patients. These nurse and social work care managers work closely with inpatient discharge planning, and ambulatory care clinics, home care providers, mental health providers, and social service organizations to support patients and their families during the gap between an acute-care hospitalization and clinic appt. Many patient questions and areas of confusion have been discovered. Roughly one third of patients called need 2 h of registered nurse time to address clinical problems. Problems include medication confusion (medication reconciliation is the major activity done by the call-back nurses); home care services that did not come; no follow-up appointment, cannot get to a clinic appointment, or do not understand why they should go; patients unsafe at home.

The post-acute call-back program has been analyzed for its effects. During a 2-year period that was specifically evaluated, May 2008 to May 2010, the program handled 31,339 of 49,744 inpatient and ED Medicare discharges. Internal administrative evaluations have suggested decreased readmissions and ED visits after the program was implemented compared to before it was implemented, and similar decreased readmissions and ED visits for patients who were called compared with those who were not called.

Improving hospital discharge: Beginning in 2008, UMHS began to participate in BOOST (Better Outcomes for Older Adults Through Safe Transitions Project sponsored by the Society of Hospital Medicine) [18] and M*STAAR (Michigan – State Action on Avoidable Rehospitalizations). Both programs stress identification of patients in the hospital who are at risk for readmission after discharge, notification of patients' primary care providers of the patients' admission and discharge and important tests that need to be followed up, and provision of high quality discharge instructions and teaching to patients and their caregivers prior to discharge. Although not directly targeted to the PGPD, this program facilitates communication between the hospital discharging physicians and nurses, and the call-back program and sub-acute program.

Sub-acute Nursing Home (NH) Service: Discharge process redesign and frail elder programs (see below) coordinate with the UMHS sub-acute service. In this service, begun during the second year of the PGPD, three geriatric faculty members practice full-time in five local high volume skilled nursing (sub-acute care) facilities supported by four geriatric nurse practitioners and the University of Michigan's electronic medical record in the nursing homes. This service handles about 45 % of the approximately 1,200 Medicare patients who are discharged to sub-acute facilities each year from UM Hospital. This innovative program has substantially reduced acute care length of stay for nursing home patients and had (and continues to have because like the other programs, it is ongoing) a small but measureable effect on NH readmissions to acute care hospitals [16].

Care Coordination for High-Risk, High-Cost, Complex Patients

Complex Care Coordination: Care coordination for complex Medicaid, Dual Eligible and homeless/uninsured complex patients is performed through the Complex Care Management Program (CCMP). The CCMP consists of 6.5 centrally located Complex Care Managers (nurses and social workers and two patient care advocates, see above), supported by a medical director, who provide chronic care management services to complex, high utilizing patients in vulnerable populations. Complex Care Managers work closely with multiple agencies within and outside UMHS, including visiting nurses, medical social workers, and community health and mental health providers. The care managers undergo standardized training and use both panel management software and the EMR. Most patients are recruited into the CCMP after they are discharged from the hospital, are evaluated by the post-acute call back service (i.e., the same nurse/social work team), and are considered to be complex based on standard criteria. Physicians, social workers, and home care providers can also refer patients. We have found that identifying patients for complex care management through a hospitalization is a very efficient way to assure that care coordination resources are directed to the high risk, high cost patients who need these resources. Over time a higher proportion of complex care managers are social workers with mental health proficiency, reflecting the importance of mental and behavioral health conditions and social services in meeting the needs of complex care patients. The characteristics, operation, and outcomes of the CCMP during and after the PGPDP have been described elsewhere [17].

Palliative Care: Patients with advanced disease beyond curable interventions, or with highly complex health status, often have preferences about their care. UMHS has a multidisciplinary palliative care and hospice program begun in 2006 that reaches across the care continuum and into the community to work with patients and families to formulate and implement such highly personal care goals. This program is anchored by an accredited palliative and hospice care fellowship (among the first programs accredited in the US) with highly experienced faculty in several Medical School departments. The program includes acute care and nursing home consult services, UMHS faculty group practice members who visit local hospices to provide services to UMHS patients, and ambulatory palliative care clinics in geriatrics and oncology.

Other Relevant Infrastructure

Geriatrics Services: For many years, UMHS has had a respected and relatively large Geriatrics clinical service. The Geriatrics clinic provides primary care and care coordination for about 5,500 frail and complex elderly who need social and personal care support. The clinic features faculty geriatricians and a multidisciplinary team with social work, nursing and pharmacy, and provides educational opportunities for interdisciplinary trainees. The Geriatrics Clinic participates in the Patient Centered Medical Home Program (see below) and is co-located with Geriatric Psychiatry, and with cognitive and movement disorder neurology clinics. Complex care management is provided by four social workers. The Geriatrics clinic has strong links to the transitional care programs, to the CCMP, and to community programs. Additional programs developed by the clinical social workers include information and referral services, caregiver and patient counseling, and links to a large day-care program for patients with cognitive impairment.

Patient-Centered Medical Home

UMHS implemented primary care redesign consistent with the Patient Centered Medical Home (PCMH) model beginning in 2008 [19]. Not all aspects of the PCMH were implemented at once in all the clinics. Full implementation took over a year and in many ways, the PCMH continues to develop. The goal of the UMHS PCMH is to empower patients to take a very active role in their own care, to learn about their conditions, to create action plans and to set goals with their provider to achieve better health.

The University of Michigan is following the joint principles of the Patient Centered Medical Home issued in 2007 by the American Academy of Family Physicians, American Academy of Pediatrics, American College of Physicians and American Osteopathic Association [19], the National Committee for Quality Assurance (NCQA), as well as the domains of function established by BCBSM.

The UMHS PCMH program includes 23 primary care clinics (all of the primary care clinics), the Geriatrics clinic, and about 196 providers. All these clinics have been designated as PCMH's under the guidelines set by BCBSM since 2009 that are consistent with, and somewhat more rigorous, than those of NCQA [20].

The domains of function established by BCBSM and met by the UMHS PCMH program include:

- An explicit working relationship with the patient and caregiver.
- Registries for chronic diseases including: diabetes, CHF, CAD, asthma, CKD and COPD. These registries offer valuable clinical information to the primary care physician and specialist to provide the patient with the best care that meets their needs.
- Leadership reports that provide feedback to leadership, health center staff and clinicians about how their patients are doing based on national benchmarks.

- Same day visit availability (30 % of schedule) and extended hours including weekends to meet the needs of the patients.
- Staff training and implementation of self-management support for patients with chronic diseases, helping patients to set self-management goals and to establish action plans to help them improve their overall health.
- Community outreach with access to a social worker as well as community resources to support the patient.
- ePrescribing.
- Coordination of care across all domains of the health care system, facilitated by the established registries, information technology and health information exchange, and with a particular focus on transitions of care from inpatient to outpatient.

The PCMH was implemented in the last year of the PGPD. Only about 50 % of attributed patients in the PGPD were in the UMHS primary care clinics. Another 25 % had primary care providers elsewhere (and may have also have seen a UMHS primary care provider), while about 25 % had no primary care at all. We do not know how primary care utilization was distributed among our market control group, but we expect that in our local area, patients do not use primary care physicians as much as in other areas of the country.

Specialty Clinic Services

Aspects of the PCMH were and still are available in major ambulatory specialty clinics at UMHS – geriatrics (as mentioned above), cardiology, endocrinology, and pulmonary. Patients in these clinics are included on chronic disease registries. Physicians receive point of care reminders for relevant chronic disease management and preventative interventions, provider feedback on clinical quality performance, and team support for care coordination and transitional care activities. Within the UMHS integrated system, the specialists are part of the ACO and many take their role of chronic disease management seriously. Some care coordination and disease management systems have historically existed within the UMHS specialty clinics often started by researchers or set up to improve disease management during the time of managed care contracts.

Key among such programs are the heart failure disease management program and the coagulation clinic. The heart failure disease management program has a medical director, nurse supported patient and caregiver care coordination and self-management support, a post-acute transitional care clinic, and a performance improvement program. The large, centralized, system wide anticoagulation monitoring program manages warfarin treatment for any patient with a UMHS physician and is housed within cardiology.

In these clinics, if a patient has a dominant chronic disease or a dominant current disease (cancer, major surgical problem, etc.), the specialist may be acting as the patient's "principle physician" either on a continuous basis (as with some cardiologists and pulmonologists) or on a time-limited basis (oncologist). This management model may have the potential, when appropriate care is known and/or incentives are aligned, to be more efficient than having a primary care physician attempt to manipulate within a "medical neighborhood" [21], and attempt to "gatekeep" or co-manage outside his/her area of expertise and potentially outside the preferences of the patient. For example, the UMHS cancer center has multiple programs for patient and caregiver support, although not as developed as the recently described cancer medical home. A recent paper described the success of UMHS in decreasing hospitalizations of cancer patients during the PGPD [13].

Quality Measurement and Performance Improvement Program

The Quality Management Program

The Quality Management Program (QMP), begun in the late 1990s in response to managed care activities of UMHS, has major responsibility for quality measurement and improvement for chronic diseases in the ambulatory setting. The QMP develops and maintains chronic disease registries, provides point-of-care reminders to clinicians, identifies gaps in care, utilizes interactive voice response technology to engage patients in self-management of depression and heart failure, maintains >25 evidence based clinical practice guidelines and >600 specialty referral guidelines, and assesses and reports on institutional, departmental and provider quality of care. In addition it receives and analyses claims data from several payers including CMS/Medicare, the state of Michigan/Medicaid, and BCBSM for multiple commercial insurance programs. The QMP has dedicated senior analysts who are adept at analyses using EMR data, healthcare system administrative data, and claims data from payers. These analyses support feedback to clinicians and clinical leaders. In addition, QMP data analysts provide analyses and reports to healthcare system leaders who are responsible for implementing care redesign interventions such as the PGPD and the PCMH, and are important resources supporting communication with payers regarding data quality, attribution issues, and financial monitoring.

Challenges Faced by UMHS in the PGPD and in Future ACO Efforts

Despite the many characteristics of the UMHS that led to success in the PGPD and could lead to success in the future, UMHS also had and still has substantial challenges as it tries to manage population health and redesign clinical care. These challenges are in part related to the fact that UMHS is an academic healthcare system. As such it has: (1) adverse patient selection that cannot fully be corrected by risk adjustment; (2) important missions of education and research in addition to clinical care; (3) high costs both because it is an academic healthcare system and it is located in a relatively high cost area. However, the design of the PGPD may have helped to counter some of these challenges.

Adverse Selection. As an Academic Healthcare System, UMHS experiences adverse selection. Patients who are referred for highly specialized care, and those with complex or severe chronic disease, often ended up in its attributed population because attribution was by plurality of outpatient costs and patients were attributed to the entire faculty group practice, not just faculty in primary care. This attribution methodology identified some patients with very high costs and pushed up the average yearly per capital cost of attributed beneficiaries. Many of UMHS's attributed Medicare beneficiaries had high costs in oncology, cardiology, or even ophthalmology, and there were more dual eligible patients than in the surrounding market area. However, among these high-risk high cost patients, there may be waste and poorly coordinated care, and therefore more opportunities to improve care efficiency.

Multiple missions: research and education. As an academic healthcare center, UMHS has many faculty members who participate in research and education as well as clinical care. Complex patients with serious illnesses are drawn to skilled, academic physicians, and many specialists may be engaged in research to define appropriate care. Therefore, high-risk high cost patients may be seeing physicians in an academic medical center who are able and willing to manage these patients efficiently. Some academic physicians may also respond to incentives related to their work in education and research rather than incentives based solely on productivity.

Medical education costs and relatively high cost market area. In an academic healthcare system direct and indirect medical education payments from Medicare contribute to costs. Other costs of academic medical centers for staffing, research support and technology can also potentially contribute to high costs of care. In addition, according to the Dartmouth Atlas, UMHS is located in a relatively high cost market area. However, the PGPD and other ACO financial models do not target lower costs, but rather, decreased growth of costs.

Conclusion

Based on UMHS characteristics as an Academic Healthcare Center, and the intersection of these characteristics with the PGPD attribution and financial methodology, it seems plausible that the success of UMHS in the PGPD was based on efficient and high quality care of high cost high-risk patients. UMHS internal analyses, CMS analyses, and published studies of the PGPD are consistent in pointing toward the hypothesis that some of the success of UMHS and the other successful participants in the PGPD may have been due to efficient care of sicker patients. Clinical and governance integration, a unified EMR, and numerous transitional care and care coordination activities are probably all very important in "bending the curve". In addition, attribution of sicker patients by attribution to the multispecialty group instead of just primary care physicians, the presence of skilled specialists and generalists who are comfortable caring for sick patients, and employed faculty physicians who are comfortable with an academic mission, may also have contributed.

Future information about the performance of the many different types of healthcare systems participating in the ACO programs may very well point to many different healthcare system configurations, including Academic Healthcare Systems, which can achieve high quality and efficient patient care.

References

1. Accountable Care Organizations (ACO). Centers for Medicare & Medicaid Services Website. http://www.cms.gov/Medicare/Medicare-Fee-for-Service-Payment/ACO/. Accessed 13 May 2014.
2. Kautter J, Pope GC, Leung M, Trisolini M, Adamache W, Smith K, Trebino D, Kaganova J, Patterson L, Berzin O, Schwartz M. Evaluation of the Medicare Physician Group Practice Demonstration final report. Research Triangle Park: RTI International; 2012.
3. Trisolini M, Kautter J, Pope GC, Bapat B, Olmsted E, Urato M. Physician Group Practice Demonstration quality measurement and reporting specifications. 2005. http://www.cms.gov/Medicare/Demonstration-Projects/DemoProjectsEvalRpts/downloads/Quality_Specs_Report.pdf. Accessed 13 May 2014.
4. Kautter J, Pope GC, Trisolini M, Grund S. Medicare Physician Group Practice Demonstration design: quality and efficiency pay-for-performance. Health Care Financ Rev. 2007;29(1):15–29.
5. Wilensky GR. Lessons from the Physician Group Practice Demonstration – a sobering reflection. N Engl J Med. 2011;365(18):1659–61.
6. Iglehart JK. Assessing an ACO prototype–Medicare's Physician Group Practice Demonstration. N Engl J Med. 2011;364(3):198–200.
7. Fisher ES, McClellan MB, Bertko J, et al. Fostering accountable health care: moving forward in Medicare. Health Aff. 2009;28(2):W219–31.
8. Sebelius K. Report to Congress: Physician Group Practice Demonstration evaluation report. 2009. http://www.cms.gov/Medicare/Demonstration-Projects/DemoProjectsEvalRpts/downloads/PGP_RTC_Sept.pdf. Accessed 13 May 2014.
9. Berwick DM. Making good on ACOs' promise – the final rule for the Medicare Shared Savings Program. N Engl J Med. 2011;365(19):1753–6.
10. Pope GC, Kautter J, Ellis RP, et al. Risk adjustment of Medicare capitation payments using the CMS-HCC model. Health Care Financ Rev. 2004;25(4):119–41.
11. Physician Quality Reporting System (Physician Quality Reporting or PQRS) formerly known as the Physician Quality Reporting Initiative (PQRI). Centers for Medicare & Medicaid Services Website. http://www.cms.gov/Medicare/Quality-Initiatives-Patient-Assessment-Instruments/pqrs/index.html. Accessed 13 May 2014.
12. Colla CH, Wennberg DE, Meara E, et al. Spending differences associated with the Medicare Physician Group Practice Demonstration. JAMA J Am Med Assoc. 2012;308(10):1015–23.
13. Colla CH, Lewis VA, Gottlieb DJ, Fisher ES. Cancer spending and accountable care organizations: evidence from the Physician Group Practice Demonstration. Healthcare. 2013;1(3–4):100–7.
14. University of Michigan Health System. http://www.med.umich.edu/. Accessed 13 May 2014.
15. Stiles RA, Mick SS, Wise CG. The logic of transaction cost economics in health care organization theory. Health Care Manag Rev. 2001;26(2):85–92.
16. Joshi DK, Bluhm RA, Malani PN, Fetyko S, Denton T, Blaum CS. The successful development of a subacute care service associated with a large academic health system. J Am Med Dir Assoc. 2012;13(6):564–7.
17. Williams BC, Paik JL, Haley LL, Grammatico GM. Centralized care management support for "high utilizers" in primary care practices at an academic medical center. Care Manag J. 2014;15(1):26–33.

18. Project BOOST: better outcomes by optimizing safe transitions. Society of Hospital Medicine Website. 2014. http://www.hospitalmedicine.org/AM/Template.cfm?Section=Home&TEMPLATE=/CM/HTMLDisplay.cfm&CONTENTID=27659. Accessed 13 May 2014.
19. Joint Principles of the Patient-Centered Medical Home. Patient-Centered Primary Care Collaborative website. 2007. http://www.aafp.org/dam/AAFP/documents/practice_management/pcmh/initiatives/PCMHJoint.pdf. Accessed 13 May 2014.
20. Patient-Centered Medical Home Recognition. National Committee for Quality Assurance (NCQA). 2014. http://www.ncqa.org/Programs/Recognition/PatientCenteredMedicalHome PCMH.aspx. Accessed 13 May 2013.
21. Fisher ES. Building a medical neighborhood for the medical home. N Engl J Med. 2008;359(12):1202–5.

Index

A
Academic healthcare system, UMHS, 210–211
Accountable care organizations (ACOs)
  adverse selection, 211
  CMS, 147–148
  definition, 188
  description, 210
  heterogeneity, 176
  initial costs, 177
  managed care, 144
  medical education costs and relatively high cost market area, 211
  Medicare Shared Savings Program, 144
  models, 77
  Montefiore Medical Center (*see* Montefiore Medical Center)
  multiple missions, 211
  PCMHs, 188
  shared savings, 176
ACOVE. *See* Assessing Care of Vulnerable Elders (ACOVE)
Acute Care for Elderly (ACE) Units, 2
Affordable Care Act (ACA)
  and ACOs
    ACO models, 72
    Center for Medicare and Medicaid Innovation (CMMI), 71
    Medicare Shared Savings Program (MSSP), 72
    Pioneer ACO program, 72
    triple aim, Institute for Healthcare Improvement, 71–72
  chronic illness, 144
  compelling business case, 89
  competitive marketplace, 155
  cost effective care and system redesign, 156
  dual eligibles (*see* Dual eligibles)
  eligibility for Medicaid, 155
  first dollar coverage, preventive services, 155
  healthcare quality, 154–155
  healthcare services, 1
  health insurance, 154, 155
  insurance reforms, 88
  patient bill of rights, 88
  payment methods, 154
  quality of care, 155
  quality/penalizing undesirable outcomes, 155
  success, 155
Agency for Healthcare Research and Quality (AHRQ), 16, 52, 165, 166
AGS. *See* American Geriatrics Society (AGS)
AHQA. *See* American Health Quality Association (AHQA)
AHRQ. *See* Agency for Healthcare Research and Quality (AHRQ)
AMA. *See* American Medical Association (AMA)
American Geriatrics Society (AGS), 2, 101
American Health Quality Association (AHQA), 29
American Medical Association (AMA)
  claims, 107
  direct purview, 106
  and FFS program, 67
  lobbying, 107
  physician services, 106
  royalties, 107
Assessing Care of Vulnerable Elders (ACOVE), 2, 172

B

Balanced Budget Act of 1997 (BBA), 69, 101, 138, 139, 142
Beneficiary and family centered care (BFCC)
  addresses variation, 23
  physicians play, 23
  QIO work, 23, 24
  and quality improvement (QI), 22
Berenson, R.A., 140–142
Blind spots, 37
Blue Cross Blue Shield of Massachusetts (BCBS), 77

C

CAHPS program. *See* Consumer Assessment of Healthcare Providers and Systems (CAHPS) program
Canada Health Act, 89–90
Capitation
  financial alignment demonstrations, 124–126
  MSSP, 72
  PACE, 123
  SNPs, 120–121
Caragonne, 136
Care coordination
  chronic illness, 140
  efforts, 134
  fee-for-service (FFS) context, 142, 194–195
  Health Maintenance Organization (HMO), 190
  IDS, 137
  local providers, 190
  Mathematica Policy Research, 143–144
  MIPA, 190
  Montefiore IPA *vs.* CMO, 190–192
  primary care practices, 189
  providers beyond hospital walls, 189
  quality of care, 136
Care management
  ACOs (*see* Accountable care organizations (ACOs))
  EHRs, 174
  GEM, 176
  GRACE model (*see* Geriatric Resources for Assessing Care for Elders (GRACE))
  home and community-based Medicaid waivers, 180–181
  Montefiore Medical Center (*see* Montefiore Medical Center)

Care Management for High Cost Beneficiaries (CMHCB), 195
Care transitions
  communication and patient education, 7
  evidenced based models, 129
  home care, 2–3
  long-term care facility, 182
  nursing home residents, 181–182
  PCMH, 209
  TCM, 181
Case management
  channeling, 136–137
  chronic illness, 140
  components, 136
  geriatrics, 146
  high value primary care, 148
  hospitalizations, 143
  intensive, 194
  stakeholder engagement, 27–28
  types, 142
CCM. *See* Chronic care model (CCM)
Centers for Medicare and Medicaid Innovation (CMMI), 50, 71, 124, 167, 182
Centers for Medicare and Medicaid Services (CMS)
  ACA, 123
  ACOs, 72, 73, 76, 77
  analysis of national performance data, 24
  CMHCB, 195
  contract, 15
  data, 19
  estimates, 4
  FCHCO, 124
  financial alignment demonstrations, 124–127
  functions, QIOs, 15
  HCC system, 161
  innovative service delivery model, 147
  and the Joint Commission, 50
  medical case review, 21
  MSSP program, 74, 75, 205
  MUO, 125, 126
  QIO program, 15
  quality strategy 2013, 29
  requirement, 49
  State Demonstration Waiver programs, 121
  transparency of quality information, 18
  value-based purchasing programs, 20, 50
Channeling demonstration, GRACE model. *See* Geriatric Resources for Assessing Care for Elders (GRACE)
"Choosing Wisely" Initiative, ABIM, 135

Index   217

Chronic care model (CCM), 145
Chronic illness
   ACA, 144
   case management, 140
   CCM, 145
   CMS, 4
   fragmented care, 136
Clinical redesign and models of care, 204–205
CMHCB. *See* Care Management for High Cost Beneficiaries (CMHCB)
CMMI. *See* Centers for Medicare and Medicaid Innovation (CMMI)
CMS. *See* Centers for Medicare and Medicaid Services (CMS)
Coaching style, leadership, 39
COGME. *See* Council on Graduate Medical Education (COGME)
Coleman Care Transitions Program, 2
Commonwealth Fund Commission, 135
Complex care coordination, 207
Comprehensive clinical care models
   ACOs, 176–177
   concierge medicine, 178
   GRACE, 179
   hospice and palliative care, 179–180
   PACE, 178
   PCMH, 177
Comprehensive outpatient rehabilitation facilities (CORFs), 24
Consumer Assessment of Healthcare Providers and Systems (CAHPS) program, 165
CORFs. *See* Comprehensive outpatient rehabilitation facilities (CORFs)
Council on Graduate Medical Education (COGME), 101

D
DEA. *See* Drug enforcement agency licensure (DEA)
Diabetes in elderly
   and hypertension, 103
   management, 104
   in older individuals, 104
Diagnosis Related Groups (DRGs), 190
Disease management
   description, 194
   health care, 40
   hospitalizations, 143
   Oxford Health, 145
   payment, 8
   PCMH, 209
   primary care extension program, 108

   telehealth (E-health), 175
Doctor's Office Quality-Information Technology (DOQ-IT) program, 19
DRGs. *See* Diagnosis Related Groups (DRGs)
Drug enforcement agency licensure (DEA), 48
Dual eligibles
   adverse selection, 211
   care coordination challenges, 118–119
   CCMP, 207
   CMS (*see* Centers for Medicare and Medicaid Services (CMS))
   description, 117–118
   diversity, 118
   geriatric medicine and primary care principles, 127–129
   models of care, 119–123
   patients
      care management of, 204
      post-acute callback program, 206
   provisions, 124, 125

E
Efficiency
   administration, 93
   care, for patients and populations, 200
   and economy, 15
   and effectiveness, 15
   and incentives, 124
   and outcomes, 50
   physician and reimbursement, 182
   and quality, 1, 4, 15, 155, 158
   and value, 1, 4
Electronic health records (EHR)
   communication, 40
   document and retrieve, information, 173
   EHR Incentive, 76
   inefficiencies in utilization, 174
   and information technologies, 129
   nurse and social worker, 129
   opportunities and challenges, 174
   physician practices, 20
Electronic medical records (EMR)
   chronic disease registries, 203
   clinical and governance integration, unified EMR, 211
   communication, 40
   Epic EMR system, 203
   and UMHS, 202
   University of Michigan (UM), 202
Email systems, 40, 141
EMCROs. *See* Experimental Medical Care Review Organizations (EMCROs)

Emergency Medical Treatment and Labor Act (EMTALA), 15, 24
Emotional intelligence
  components, 54
  definition, 35
  empathy and social skills, 36
  physician recruitment, 44
  self-awareness, 35
Empathy, 8, 9, 35, 36, 42, 43
EMR. *See* Electronic medical records (EMR)
EMTALA. *See* Emergency Medical Treatment and Labor Act (EMTALA)
End-stage renal disease (ESRD), 188
Enhanced primary care, 128–129
Enthoven, A.C., 137, 138
ESRD. *See* End-stage renal disease (ESRD)
ESTJ. *See* Extroversion/sensing/thinking/judging (ESTJ)
Experimental Medical Care Review Organizations (EMCROs), 16
Extroversion/sensing/thinking/judging (ESTJ), 37

F
Federal Coordinated Health Care Office (FCHCO), 124
Fee-for-service (FFS)
  CMHCB, 195
  Medicare program, 194
  pioneer ACO, 195
  program, 67
Financial and legal skills, physician leaders
  antifraud laws, 56
  budgeting and designing compensation arrangements, 56
  employment law, 56
  healthcare institutions, 56
  job description, 56–62
  malpractice, 56
  Stark law, 56
Flexner report, 99
Focused professional practice evaluation (FPPE), 49
Fragmented care
  ACO, 77
  chronic illness, 136
  health care settings, 135
Frail elderly
  ACOVE, 2
  channeling, 136–137
  PACE, 149
  PQRS, 109
  sub-acute NH service, 206–207
Frailty, 123

G
GEM. *See* Geriatric evaluation and management (GEM)
Geriatric care models
  comprehensive clinical care models, 176–180
  description, 169–170
  EHR, 173–175
  GEM, 175–176
  high risk populations, 171–172
  home and community-based Medicaid waivers, 180–181
  older adults, characteristics, 170–171
  opportunities and limitations, 172–173
  telehealth (E-health), 175
  transitional care interventions, 181–182
Geriatric evaluation and management (GEM), 175–176
Geriatric fellowship programs
  board certification exam, 105
  financial incentives, 110
  geriatrician educators and leaders, development, 109
  lowest paying field, 106
  Medicare program, 101
Geriatricians. *See also* Healthcare models
  ACE and GRACE, 2
  Affordable Care Act, 1
  charge, hospital discharge planners, 134
  consultant, 129
  development, 100
  financial incentives, cost reduction in hospital utilization, 106
  and geriatric health care professionals, 103
  healthcare infrastructure, 109
  job satisfaction, 111
  leader and educator, 109, 110
  median salary, 106
  NICHE, 3
  older individuals, 103
  PACE and ACOVE, 2
  physicians, 1
  policy and program development, 104
  PQRS metrics, 109
  primary care, 134
  and primary care physicians, 106–109
  QIO, 28
  skill set, 104
  training, 112
  in United States, 105
  US healthcare, 1
Geriatric medicine
  board certification, 105, 106
  career, 112
  clinical management, older adults, 112

Index 219

development, 102, 104
GeriMed philosophy of care, 102, 141
internal medicine, 104
physician workforce, 99
pragmatic and manageable approach, 110
primary care geriatrics, 109
and primary care principles, 127–129
principles, 110
socioeconomic issues, 102
Geriatric Resources for Assessing Care for Elders (GRACE)
  ACOs (*see* Accountable care organizations (ACOs))
  BBA of 1997, 139
  case management (*see* Case management)
  CCM, 145
  channeling, 136–137
  'Choosing Wisely' Initiative, 135
  chronic illness, 140
  description, 2, 133
  GeriMed of America, 138
  health care delivery system fragmentation, 135–136
  hospital utilization rates, 133–134
  integrated delivery system (IDS), 137
  interdisciplinary teams, 2
  intervention, 146–147
  mathematica policy research, 143–144
  Medicare reimbursement system, 140–142
  Oxford Health, 145
  PACE, 148–149
  payment and delivery systems, 134–135
  primary care physicians (PCP) office, 128
  Senior Care of Colorado, 139–140
Geriatrics
  AGS, 101
  APRN, 111
  board certification, 105
  and cardiology, 206
  career, 101, 112
  care models, 172–173
  definition, 103
  development, 100, 102
  education, 109, 110
  evaluation and management, 175–176
  fellowship program, 101, 105, 106, 109, 110
  GME financing, 105
  GRACE, 2, 179
  health care professionals, 103
  healthcare workforce, 111
  intervention, 171, 172
  lack of training, 146
  medical care approach, 148

  medical education, 102
  medicine (*see* Geriatric medicine)
  pharmacy and psychiatry, 28, 111
  and primary care, 107, 109
  and primary care providers, 127–129
  principles, 146
  residency positions, 135
  services
    PCMH model, 208–209
    primary care and care coordination, 208
  syndromes, 103, 170
  training, 111
  UMHS, 209
  United States, 101, 102
GeriMed Philosophy of Care, 102, 138, 139, 141
Gerogeriatrics, 103
GME. *See* Graduate medical education (GME)
GRACE. *See* Geriatric Resources for Assessing Care for Elders (GRACE)
Graduate medical education (GME)
  Council, 101
  Federal support, 104
  funds, 111
  government financing, 105
  Medicare Trust Fund, 101
  primary care geriatrics, 109
  program, 101
  public funding, 100–101
  redistribution, 108
  structure, 101, 110, 113
  subsidies and reimbursement incentives, 112
  subsidization, 105
Group Health Cooperative of Puget Sound, 68

H

HCC system. *See* Hierarchical Condition Category (HCC) system
HCQII. *See* Health Care Quality Improvement Initiative (HCQII)
HCQIP. *See* Health Care Quality Improvement Program (HCQIP)
Health and Human Services (HHS), 29, 72, 95, 166
Healthcare, communication and coordination of care, 87
Healthcare effectiveness data and information set (HEDIS), 50, 201
Healthcare models
  collaborators and innovators, 4
  Institute for Healthcare Improvement, 4

Healthcare models (*cont.*)
   national variation, Medicare spending, 4, 5
   OASI, DI and HI trust fund ratios, 5, 6
   total health expenditure per capita, 3
   UN World Population Prospectus, 5, 6
Health Care Quality Improvement Initiative (HCQII), 17
Health Care Quality Improvement Program (HCQIP), 17
Healthcare reform, 205
Healthcare Research and Quality (AHRQ), 16, 52, 165, 166
Healthcare workforce
   geriatric, 111
   training of physicians and number of geriatricians., 111
   in United States, 99
Health insurance, 153
Health Maintenance Organization (HMO), 67, 190
HEDIS. *See* Healthcare effectiveness data and information set (HEDIS)
HHS. *See* Health and Human Services (HHS)
Hierarchical Condition Category (HCC) system, 161, 201
High value primary care, 148
HMO. *See* Health Maintenance Organization (HMO)
HMO Act of 1973, 68
Home and community-based Medicaid waivers, 180–181
Hospice and palliative care, 179–180
Household economies, 153
HR676 (United States Congress)
   clerical, administrative and billing personnel, 93
   National Board of Universal Quality and Access, 93
   patients, freedom of choice, 92
   pharmaceuticals, medical supplies and assistive equipment, 93
   private physicians and clinics, 92
   single payer, health care budgeting, 93
   single payer system, 93
HYVET study, 104

I
IDS. *See* Integrated delivery system (IDS)
Iglehart, J.K., 140–141
Ignatz L.N., 101
IHI. *See* Institute for Healthcare Improvement (IHI)
Improvement, quality

   BPCI, 182
   clinical quality improvement program, 204
   coaching style, 39
   CQI, 133
   definition, 50
   and financial advantages, 177
   health-related quality of life, 129
   IHI, 51, 71
   institute for healthcare improvement, 4
   INTERACT, 2, 181–182
   measurement, 163
   QIO (*see* Quality Improvement Organization (QIO))
   quality and billing documentation, 174
   quality and safety committees, 10
   quality measurement and performance improvement program, 210
   and quality measures, 176
   and role in evaluation, 157
   urban safety-net hospital, 34
Independent physician associations (IPA), 40, 48, 190–192
Innovation, healthcare
   ACO's, 8
   cost-conscious care, 8
   hospital acquired conditions, 7
   hospital safety programs, 7
   Patient Centered Medical Home, The, 7
   physicians, 8
Institute for Healthcare Improvement (IHI), 51
Integrated care
   financial incentives, 130
   GRACE model, 148
   Mathematica Policy Research, 144
   PCMH, 128
   SNPs, 120–121
Integrated delivery system (IDS)
   ACO, 8
   care coordination mode, 137
   Montefiore's, 189
   MSSP, 72
Integrated financing. *See* Medicare-Medicaid financial alignment demonstration
INTERACT. *See* Interventions to Reduce Acute Care Transfers (INTERACT)
Interprofessional teams, 128
Interventions to Reduce Acute Care Transfers (INTERACT), 2–3, 19, 23, 181–182
Introversion/sensing/thinking/judging (ISTJ), 37
IPA. *See* Independent physician associations (IPA)
ISTJ. *See* Introversion/sensing/thinking/judging (ISTJ)

Index

J
Journal of the American Medical Association (JAMA), 25

L
LAN. *See* Learning and action network (LAN)
LANE. *See* Local area networks for excellence (LANE)
Leadership
  ACO, 157
  advice, 37–38
  change, 9
  definition, 34–35
  emotional intelligence, 35–36
  functions, 9–10
  and management skills, 104
  persistence, 9
  personality types, 36–37
  physician
    lead and manage system, 33
    managing and expectations, 39–41
    skills (*see* Physician leadership skills)
  QIOs, 18
  risk tolerance, 9
  styles, 38–39
  trust, 9
Learning and action network (LAN), 24, 25
Local area networks for excellence (LANE), 28
Low volume providers, 49

M
Managed Care (MCARE). *See also* Care management
  BCBSM, 204
  and cost pressures, 68–69
  enrollment, 126
  health maintenance organizations (HMOs), 144
  Medicare advantages, 120
  non-integrated, 120
  patient alignment and engagement, 73–74
  provider-based health-care plans, 203
  UMHS providers, 203
  vs. Medicare FFS, 67–68
  Wisconsin Partnership Program, 121
Mathematica policy research
  case and disease management, 142–143
  hospitalizations, 143–144
MCARE and Medicare, cost pressure and expansion
  Balanced Budget Act of 1997 (BBA), 69
  capitated payments, 68
  HMO plans, 69
  managed care enrollment rate, decline in, 69
  Medicare advantages, 69
  Medicare Modernization Act (MMA, 2003), 69
  outsized cost growth, reasons, 68
  payment reforms, 68
  right-size payments, 69
Medicaid, geriatric care models. *see* Geriatric care models
Medical home model. *See* Patient Centered Medical Home (PCMH)
Medical specialty society, 166
Medicare
  ACOs, 176–177, 201
  advantages, 139, 155, 160
  beneficiaries, 15–16, 20–24, 153
  BFCC QIO work, 24
  CMMI, 182
  CMS (*see* Centers for Medicare and Medicaid Services (CMS))
  coordinated care, 142
  cost pressures, Medicare and Managed care, 68–69
  end stage renal disease, 154
  fee-for-service care, 18
  FFS populations, 194
  FFS *vs.* managed care history and payment mechanics, 67–68
  geriatric care models (*see* Geriatric care models)
  GRACE model (*see* Geriatric Resources for Assessing Care for Elders (GRACE))
  and health care costs, 104
  health care legislation, 92
  healthcare system and country, 154
  HMO's, 138
  hospice and palliative care, 179–180
  hospitalizations and re-hospitalizations, 25
  legislation, 100
  limitations, 91
  and Medicaid coordination, 117–130
  and Medicaid programs, 17
  PACE, 178
  patients, 105
  payment, 107
  pioneer and MSSP ACO programs, 73–77
  private insurance companies, 90–91
  program, 66–67
  PRO program, 16, 18
  public confidence, 90
  reimbursement, 107

Medicare (cont.)
    RUC, 106–107
    shared savings program, 144
    "single-payer" system, 92
    Social Security Administration, The, 90
    success/failure, 154
    Trust Fund, 100–101
Medicare and Medicaid coordination. *See* Dual eligibles
Medicare Coordinated Care Demonstration, 142, 145
Medicare FFS *vs.* Managed Care, payment mechanics
    Group Health Cooperative of Puget Sound, 68
    group practices, 67
    Health Maintenance Organizations (HMO), 67
    HMO Act of 1973, 67, 68
    Managed care, Medicare program, 67
    Medicare program, 67
    prepaid health plans, concept of, 67
    prepayment demonstrations, 68
Medicare for All, 92, 93
Medicare-Medicaid financial alignment demonstration
    capitation, 124
    clinical programs, 126
    consumer concerns, 126–127
    fee-for-service model, 124
    insurance companies, 126
Medicare Modernization Act (MMA, 2003), 69
Medicare Payment Advisory Commission (MedPAC), 70, 77
Medicare Pioneer and MSSP ACO programs, features
    alternative quality contracting (AQC) model, 77
    care coordination, 77
    financial model, 74–75
    Medicare-enrolled Tax identification number (TIN), 73
    patient alignment and engagement, 73–74
    performance-based payment contracts, 75
    physician payment, 75–76
    Pioneer ACO program, 73
    population-based payments, 75
    provider participation and length of programs
    quality monitoring
        Electronic Health Record (EHR) Incentive, 76
        metrics, categories, 76
        Physician Quality Reporting System programs, 76
    risk levels, 75
Medicare Program, history of, 66–67
Medicare risk adjustment
    BBA of 1997, 139
    episode treatment group, 162
    expenditures, 161
    PGPD, 200, 201
    process measures, 157
    Senior Care of Colorado, 139–140
    SES, 163
Medicare Trust Fund, 5, 6, 15, 16, 78, 100, 101
MedWise Center, 138, 139
Memorandum of understanding (MUO), 125, 126
MIPA. *See* Montefiore Integrated Provider Association (MIPA)
Models of care
    chronic illness, 140
    demonstration projects, 123
    geriatric, 2
    Medicaid services, 119
    Medicare advantage, 120
    PACE, 121–123
    physician behavior, 141
    PPACA, 20–21
    Senior Care of Colorado, 139
    SNPs, 120–121
    Social Security Act, 119
    waiver programs, 121
Montefiore Care Guidance Program
    approach, 193–194
    CMO structure, 193
    staff, 192
Montefiore Care Management Organization (CMO)
    care guidance approach, 193–194
    physician leaders and providers, 192
    population management timeline, 191, 192
    structure, 193
    vs. IPA, 190, 191
Montefiore Integrated Provider Association (MIPA), 190
Montefiore Medical Center
    care coordination (*see* Care coordination)
    hospital and community-based programs, 189
    integrated delivery system, 189
    Montefiore Care Guidance Program, 191–194
MUO. *See* Memorandum of understanding (MUO)
Myers–Briggs type indicator, 36–37, 43, 53

Index

N
NAS. *See* Next Accreditation System (NAS)
National Council on Quality Assurance (NCQA), 50, 166, 208
National health program, 86
National Quality Forum (NQF), 166, 167
National Quality Strategy (NQS)
  ACA, 166–167
  AHRQ, 166
  electronic records, 166
  Measures Application Partnership, 167
  National Priorities Partnership, 167
  2013 progress report, 167–168
  project evaluations, 167
NCQA. *See* National Council on Quality Assurance (NCQA)
Next Accreditation System (NAS), 110
NICHE. *See* Nurses Improving the Care of HealthSystem Elders (NICHE)
NQF. *See* National Quality Forum (NQF)
NQS. *See* National Quality Strategy (NQS)
Nurses Improving the Care of HealthSystem Elders (NICHE), 3
Nursing homes
  care transitions, 2–3
  channeling, 137
  CMS, 18
  home-and community-based programs, 180–181
  INTERACT, 19, 181–182
  PACE, 2, 121, 148–149, 178
  QIOs, 15, 25
  residents, transitional care, 181–182
  SNPs, 120

O
Office of Inspector General (OIG), 104
Omnibus Budget Reconciliation Act of 1989 (OBRA), 106
Ongoing professional practice evaluation (OPPE), 49
Oxford Health, 145

P
PACE. *See* Program of all-inclusive care for the elderly (PACE)
Palliative care, 207
Patient Centered Medical Home (PCMH)
  BCBSM, 204, 208–209
  empower patients, 208
  Medicare and Medicaid services, 128
  UMHS, 203, 208

Patient Protection and Affordable Care Act (PPACA), 20–21
Patient Safety Organizations (PSOs), 52
PCIP. *See* Primary Care Incentive Program (PCIP)
PCMH. *See* Patient Centered Medical Home (PCMH)
PDSA cycle. *See* Plan-Do-Study-Act (PDSA) cycle
Pediatrics
  American Academy of Pediatrics, 208
  board certification, 100
  in childhood, 102
  and family physicians, 157
  geriatrics, 100
  growth, 100
  internal medicine, surgery and obstetrics, 100
  and social medicine, 189
  twentieth century, 100
Peer Review Improvement Act of 1982, 16
Peer Review Organization (PRO)
  CMS rename, 18
  definition, 17
  local projects, 18
  Medicare Trust Fund directly, 16
  quality monitoring and review activities, 16
  SOW contract cycle, 16
  utilization and quality control, 16
Performance evaluation, physician leadership skills
  administrative, 55
  appraisal, 54
  clinical activities, 54
  communicating, 54
  driving performance, 52–53
  educational activities, 54
  employee engagement, 55
  feedback sandwich method, 55
  open-ended subjective comments, 54
  personal, 55
  quality metrics, 53
  research (basic/clinical), 54
  RVUs, 53
  targets/characteristics, 53
  technical data, 53
  thinking-judging (TJ) type personalities, 53
PGPD. *See* Physician Group Practice Demonstration (PGPD)
Physician, Action Quality Improvement Organizations
  affiliations, 28

Physician, Action Quality Improvement
    Organizations (*cont.*)
  BFCC work, 23–24
  community/organizations working, 25
  education and research, 16
  heart disease, diabetes and preventive care, 17
  leadership, 21
    lead and manage system, 33
    managing and expectations, 39–41
    skills (*see* Physician leadership skills)
  Medicare's inception, 16
  PLN, 29
  practices, 20
  physician associate clinical coordinators, 18
  PROs, 16
  QIO, 18–20
  role, QIO, 25–26
  skills, 26–27
  stakeholder relationships, 17
Physician Group Practice Demonstration (PGPD)
  and EMR (*see* Electronic medical records (EMR))
  Medicare Shared Savings Program, 200
  Pioneer demonstration, 200
  retrospective patient assignment, 200–201
  risk adjustment, 201
  structural and organizational characteristics, 200
  University of Michigan (UM), 200
Physician leadership network (PLN), 29
Physician leadership skills
  credential and privilege, 48–49
  description, 43–44
  financial and legal, 56–62
  management, 43
  negotiation
    ACO environment, 47
    distributive, 47
    distributive and integrative, 46
    integrative/cooperative, 47
    networks grow and market share, 46–47
    preparation, 47
    prior relationship/hidden issues, 47
    sign-off, 48
  performance evaluation, 52–55
  quality of care, 50–51
  recruitment
    ACO/capitated environment, 44
    agencies, 46
    clinical positions, 45–46
    curriculum vitae, 46
    job description, 45, 46
    nonverbal communication, 46
    objectives, 44
    primary care and specialists, 44
    and professional staff, 44
    search, 45
    strategic planning and negotiation, 44
    type and level, 45
    voluntary/staff model, 45
  systems of care and patient safety, 51–52
Physician leaders, quality improvement and safety committees, 10
Physician Quality Reporting System (PQRS), 21, 109, 164, 166–168, 200
Physician, role of
  accountable care, 40
  coaching, 43
  communication, 40
  diabetic adult, 40
  diagnosis and treatment services, 39
  electronic medical records (EMRs), 40
  email systems, 40
  employment/associated (independent physician association, IPA) model, 40
  employ patients/consumer groups, 41
  episodic care, 40
  face-to-face encounter, 39
  generational expectations, 40
  honest examination, 43
  intellectual challenges, 42
  interpersonal relationships, 42
  leadership roles, 42
  leadership training programs, 43
  mentorship, 43
  Myers–Briggs test and feedback, 43
  own intellectual challenges, 42
  responsibility, 43
  success/failure, 41–42
  training, 39
  web-based communication, 40
Physician workforce
  aging population, 99
  Balanced Budget Act of 1997, 101
  direct and indirect support, GME, 101
  health care, population, 101
  lack of primary care physicians and geriatricians., 109
  Medicare legislation, 100
  older population, 101
Pioneer ACO program, 72, 73. *See also* Fee-for-service (FFS)
Plan-Do-Study-Act (PDSA) cycle, 17
Player-coach model, 41–42

Index

PLN. *See* Physician leadership network (PLN)
Post-acute callback program
    acute and ambulatory care settings, 205
    consultant pharmacist and home care service provider, 206
    internal administrative evaluations, 206
PPACA. *See* Patient Protection and Affordable Care Act (PPACA)
PQRS. *See* Physician Quality Reporting System (PQRS)
Primary Care Incentive Program (PCIP), 107
PRO. *See* Peer Review Organization (PRO)
Professional Standards Review Organizations (PSROs), 16
Program of all-inclusive care for the elderly (PACE)
    community providers, 122
    cost of care, 149
    dementia, 122
    description, 2
    frail seniors, 2
    Medicaid rate, 123
    nursing, 121
    quality of care, 149
Prostate Cancer in the elderly, 103
Provider-based accountability
    "extended hospital staff", 71
    managed care criticisms, 71
    Medicare Payment Advisory Commission (MedPAC), 70
    non-HMO/managed care models, 70
    Physician Group Practice (PGP) demonstration, 70
    "predominant care physician", 71
    Sustainable Growth Rate (SGR) system, 70
    virtual organizational structures, 71
PSOs. *See* Patient Safety Organizations (PSOs)
PSROs. *See* Professional Standards Review Organizations (PSROs)

Q

QA. *See* Quality assurance (QA)
QAPI. *See* Quality assurance and performance improvement (QAPI)
QIO. *See* Quality Improvement Organization (QIO)
QMP. *See* Quality Management Program (QMP)
Quality
    AHRQ, 4, 165
    attributes, 159
    and care coordination, 120
    and cost, 146

    CQI, 133
    and efficiency, 155
    floor quality performance rate, 164
    healthcare, 50–51, 154
    and health insurance, 155
    improving, 147, 181
    measurement (*see* Quality measurement)
    minor burn care, 160
    monitoring, 76
    NCQA, 166, 208
    NQS, 166–168
    outcomes, 71
    payment, 154
    and penalizing undesirable outcomes, 155
    performance measurement, 166
    PQRS, 164, 200
    QIO (*see* Quality Improvement Organization (QIO))
    and satisfaction, 71, 154
    transparency, 1
Quality assurance (QA), 22, 23
Quality assurance and performance improvement (QAPI), 20, 25
Quality Improvement Organization (QIO)
    AHRQ, 16
    capabilities, 21–22
    CMS, 15, 18, 19
    contract cycles, 17
    contract with CMS, 7
    description, 15
    DOQ-IT, 19
    EMCROs, 16
    EMTALA, 15
    HCQII, 17
    HCQIP, 17
    INTERACT, 19
    Medicare, 15–17
    PDSA cycle, 17
    Peer Review Improvement Act of 1982, 16
    PPACA, 20–21
    PROs, 16, 17
    PSROs, 16
    role of physician, 25–26
    skills, 26–27
    SOWs (*see* Scope/statement of works (SOWs))
    stakeholder engagement, 27–28
    state, 7
    trade association, 29
    work of
        BFCC, 22–24
        casebased approach, 23
        communities, 25
        JAMA, 24–25
        LANs, 24, 25

Quality Improvement Organization (*cont.*)
    Medicare beneficiaries, 22
    QAPI, 25
    QI and QA, 22
    quality of care, 22
    setting-based approach, 23
    systems and process, 22–23
Quality Management Program (QMP), 210
Quality measurement
    ACA, 166
    adjustments, 161–163
    attributes, 159
    denominators, 159
    diabetes, 156
    domains of health care quality, 158
    improvement and performance, 163–164
    Medicare pioneer ACO program, 164
    NQF, 166
    NQS, 158
    and outcomes, 156, 157
    performance, 166
    and performance, 203
    and performance improvement program, 210
    population size and attribution, 160–161
    PQRS, 164
    prevention, acute care/chronic disease management, 158
    process, 157
    provider types and population subsets, 165–166
    and selection criteria, 156
    structure, 157
    testing process, 163
    thresholds, 164–165
    unit of, 158
    value based payment language, 160

R
Re-hospitalizations. *See* Transitional care model (TCM)
Relative Value Scale Update Committee (RUC)
    and AMA, 107
    definition, 106
    physicians, 106
    primary care, 107
Resource-based relative value scale (RBRVS), 106
Riopelle, Dr. Jim, 138
RUC. *See* Relative Value Scale Update Committee (RUC)

S
Scope/statement of works (SOWs)
    beneficiary protection, 19
    CMS, 19
    contract cycle, 16, 17
    definition, 16
    HCQII, 17
    incremental improvements on quality metrics, 18–19
    individual PROs, 18
    national performance measurement, 18
    PROs' mandatory quality monitoring and review activities, 16
    QIO contracts, 15
    QIO performance, 18
    quality improvement, 17
    reducing inappropriate hospital admissions, 16
    support providers, 21
Self-awareness, 36
Self-management skills, 35–36
Self-regulation, 36
Senior Care of Colorado, 139, 141, 148
SES. *See* Socio-economic status (SES)
SGR. *See* Sustainable growth rate (SGR)
Single payer system
    American health care system, 83
    Brisdelle, 87
    cost-related problems accessing care, 84
    CT scans and MRI exams, 85
    paroxetine formulation, 86
    physicians, 84–85
    price discrimination and cost shifting, 95
    pricing and bureaucracy, 86
    single public/quasi-public agency, 92
Skills
    empathy and social, 35, 36
    management, 104
    physician leaders (*see* Physician leadership skills)
    QIO
        analytic skills, 26
        communication, 27
        creativity, 26–27
        education, 27
        networking, 27
        QI tools and techniques, 26
        systems and critical thinking, 26
        teamwork, 26
    self-management, 35
SNPs. *See* Special needs plans (SNPs)
Social skills, 35, 36
Socio-economic status (SES), 163

SOWs. *See* Scope/statement of works (SOWs)
Special needs plans (SNPs), 120–121
Specialty clinic services, 209–210
Stakeholder engagement, 27–28
Stark law, 56
Styles, leadership
    coaching, 39
    crisis situation, 38
    democracy, 39
    description, 38
    healthcare organizations, 38
    political dictators/fascists, 38
    positive and negative, 38
    vision, 38
Sub-acute nursing home (NH) service, 206–207
Success/failure, physician leaders, 41–42
Sustainable growth rate (SGR), 70, 161

T
TCM. *See* Transitional care model (TCM)
Telehealth (E-Health), 175
Telemedicine, 175
Thinking and judging (TJ), 37
"Three layer cake" of programs, Social Security Act amendments (1965), 67

Trade association, 29
Transitional care model (TCM)
    interventions
        long-term care facility, 182
        nursing home residents, 181–182
        TCM, 181
    programs
        acute and ambulatory care settings, 205
        hospital discharge improvement, 206
        post-acute callback program, 206–207
        sub-acute nursing home (NH) service, 206–207

U
U.S. Department of Health and Human Services, 72

V
Value based purchasing, 7, 20, 50, 53, 165, 167

W
Wagner, E.H., 145
Warren, M., 102
Web-based communication, 40

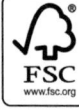

MIX
Papier aus verantwortungsvollen Quellen
Paper from responsible sources
FSC® C105338

If you have any concerns about our products,
you can contact us on
ProductSafety@springernature.com

In case Publisher is established outside the EU,
the EU authorized representative is:
**Springer Nature Customer Service Center GmbH
Europaplatz 3, 69115 Heidelberg, Germany**

Printed by Libri Plureos GmbH
in Hamburg, Germany